EXECUTIVE FUNCTIONS

Selected Works by Russell A. Barkley

For more information, visit the author's website: *www.russellbarkley.org*

FOR PROFESSIONALS

ADHD in Adults: What the Science Says
Russell A. Barkley, Kevin R. Murphy, and Mariellen Fischer

FOR GENERAL READERS

Taking Charge of ADHD, Revised Edition:
The Complete, Authoritative Guide for Parents
Russell A. Barkley

Your Defiant Child: Eight Steps to Better Behavior
Russell A. Barkley

Your Defiant Teen: 10 Steps to Resolve Conflict
and Rebuild Your Relationship
Russell A. Barkley and Arthur L. Robin with Christine M. Benton

ADULT ASSESSMENT SCALES

Barkley Adult ADHD Rating Scale–IV (BAARS-IV)
Russell A. Barkley

Barkley Deficits in Executive Functioning Scale (BDEFS for Adults)
Russell A. Barkley

Barkley Functional Impairment Scale (BFIS for Adults)
Russell A. Barkley

CHILD ASSESSMENT SCALES

Barkley Deficits in Executive Functioning Scale—
Children and Adolescents (BDEFS-CA)
Russell A. Barkley

Barkley Functional Impairment Scale—
Children and Adolescents (BFIS-CA)
Russell A. Barkley

EXECUTIVE FUNCTIONS

What They Are, How They Work, and Why They Evolved

RUSSELL A. BARKLEY

THE GUILFORD PRESS
New York   London

©2012 The Guilford Press
A Division of Guilford Publications, Inc.
370 Seventh Avenue, Suite 1200, New York, NY 10001
www.guilford.com

Printed in the United States of America

This book is printed on acid-free paper.

Last digit is print number: 9 8 7 6 5 4

Library of Congress Cataloging-in-Publication Data

Barkley, Russell A., 1949–
  Executive functions : what they are, how they work, and why they evolved /
Russell A. Barkley.
    p. cm.
  Includes bibliographical references and index.
  ISBN 978-1-4625-0535-7 (hardcover : alk. paper)
  1. Neuropsychological tests.   I. Title.
  RC386.6.N48B376 2012
  616.8′0475—dc23
                                            2012005366

For Pat, Steve, Ken, Laura, and Liam

About the Author

Russell A. Barkley, PhD, ABPP, is Clinical Professor of Psychiatry and Pediatrics at the Medical University of South Carolina. Dr. Barkley has published numerous books and five assessment scales, plus more than 260 scientific articles and book chapters on ADHD, executive functioning, and childhood defiance. He is also the editor of the newsletter *The ADHD Report*. A frequent conference presenter and speaker who is widely cited in the national media, he is past president of the Section on Clinical Child Psychology (the former Division 12) of the American Psychological Association, and of the International Society for Research in Child and Adolescent Psychopathology.

About the Author

Russell A. Barkley, PhD, ABPP, ABCN, is Clinical Professor of Psychiatry at the Virginia Treatment Center for Children and Virginia Commonwealth University School of Medicine. Dr. Barkley has worked with children, adolescents, and families since the 1970s and is the author of numerous bestselling books for both professionals and the public, including *Taking Charge of ADHD* and *Your Defiant Child*. He has also published six assessment scales and more than 280 scientific articles and book chapters on ADHD, executive functioning, and childhood defiance, and is editor of the newsletter *The ADHD Report*. A frequent conference presenter and speaker who is widely cited in the national media, Dr. Barkley is past president of the Section on Clinical Child Psychology (the former Division 12) of the American Psychological Association (APA), and of the International Society for Research in Child and Adolescent Psychopathology. He is a recipient of awards from the American Academy of Pediatrics and the APA, among other honors. His website is *www.russellbarkley.org*.

Contents

1

Problems with the Concept of Executive Functioning

The basis for the concept of executive functioning (EF) arose in the 1840s in the initial efforts by scientists to understand the functions of the frontal lobes generally and the prefrontal cortex (PFC) specifically (Harlow, 1848, 1868; Luria, 1966). Indeed, the concept predates the term "EF" by more than 120 years. The concept of EF was at first defined by default as what the prefrontal lobes do (Pribram, 1973, 1976); they are, as Pribram said, the executive brain. The term "EF" came out of these earlier efforts to understand the neuropsychological functions mediated by the prefrontal or premotor regions of the brain. This history has led to a conflating of the term "EF" with the functions of the PFC and vice versa.

Over time, this conflation has led to a circularity of reasoning in that the functions of the PFC are said to be EF while EF is then defined back to the functions of the PFC. It has also led to a slippage in the discourse on EF between two separate levels of analysis (Denckla, 1996). One is the neuropsychological level involving thought (cognition), emotion, and verbal or motor action (behavior); the other is the neuroanatomical level involving the localization of those neuropsychological functions to specific regions of the brain and their physiological activity. But EF is not exclusively a function of the PFC given that the PFC has various networks of connections to other cortical and subcortical regions as well as to the basal ganglia, amygdala and limbic system, and cerebellum (Denckla, 1996; Fuster, 1989, 1997; Luria, 1966; Nigg & Casey, 2005; Stuss & Benson, 1986). The PFC may well engage in certain neuropsychological functions that would not be considered to fall under the umbrella of EF,

1

such as simple or automatic sensory–motor activities, speech, and olfactory identification, to name just a few.

Thus, despite an extensive history concerning the nature of EF and of the functions of the PFC, several significant problems continue to exist in the definition of the term "EF," its conceptualization, and its measurement. EF is a term describing psychological functions and is therefore a construct at the psychological level of analysis. If our understanding of EF is to advance, the concept of EF and its nature must be defined separately and specifically at the psychological level without reference to the neurological level being an essential part of that definition. Such a cross-referencing of levels is of interest to neuropsychology in determining what specific brain regions engage in what specific functions. But this activity requires that we have such functions properly defined at the psychological level first before we can determine what brain networks give rise to that psychological function. If EF and its larger purposes in human life are not well defined and developed, only confusion can reign at the neurological level as one searches for the neural networks that supposedly underlie a vaguely defined and poorly crafted psychological construct, perhaps in vain.

This book was written to address four related problems that currently exist in the concept of EF. First, there is neither a consensus definition of EF nor an explicit operational definition of the term that can simply, clearly, and efficiently determine which human mental functions can be considered executive in nature and which ones cannot be so classified. Simply put, What is EF? When definitions are too general or vague, as is EF, they leave considerable opportunity for misinterpretation as well as for including within the term's conceptual realm excessive semantic baggage that would easily have been pared away had the definition had greater clarity and precision.

The first problem leads to the second. How is EF to be assessed? If the term is not defined operationally then anything goes; any measure or test can be declared to be executive in nature by mere assertion alone or through its alignment with any of 33 constructs attributed to it (Eslinger, 1996). As a case in point, my colleagues and I declared the Simon game to be a test of EF in one of our studies on adult attention-deficit/hyperactivity disorder (ADHD) (Murphy, Barkley, & Bush, 2001). This game requires one to replicate increasingly longer sequences of musical notes by depressing keys corresponding to each note. We asserted that this was a test of EF because it assessed nonverbal working memory and that it was similar to that of digit span in the verbal domain; this assertion went unquestioned in reviews of our paper. Granted, working memory has been defined as holding information in mind that is used to guide subsequent behavior, and this game seems to fulfill that definition. But then why is holding information in mind (working memory) itself an executive function? As a consequence of lack of definitional clarity, many tests and measures have been declared to be executive functioning tests without much basis for challenge. And so we cycle back to the first problem—the absence of an operational definition of EF, which then spawns the use of any variation of a test a researcher or clinician wishes to use to measure EF. To make the tautology complete, models of EF are then empirically developed based on tests of EF. Yet if there are problems in the choice of what measures assess EF, then these problems carry forward to create problems in the theories constructed upon them. Not the least of these problems is that of method variance—the theory will largely reflect the types of tests used to construct the model rather than being based on conceptual clarity and operational definition.

This state of affairs is actually related to a third larger problem this book intends to address: the lack of a coherent theory of EF. Theories are not just constructs, but mechanisms, which is to say explanations of relationships among constructs. They address the questions of How does EF work? or What does it do? Without a coherent theory of EF, constructs have multiplied to the extent that 33 or more have been claimed to be involved in this "metaconstruct" or umbrella term (Eslinger, 1996). The relationships among these various constructs have only been vaguely explained. For instance, are response inhibition and planning and problem solving related to each other? If so, in what way are they interactive? If not, why not, given that they have all been considered to be EF? So they must have some relationship to each other or else combining them under the umbrella construct of EF is nonsensical. If our goals are precision of thinking and definition as well as utility of prediction, this situation is patently unacceptable. Prediction requires explanation or understanding, and that requires propositions about how things relate to each other. Listing a set of constructs that are presumed to make up an umbrella, family, or metaconstruct will not suffice. There must be some operational definition as to what makes that list executive in nature and just how the constructs being labeled as EF relate to each other. In the absence of such an explanation, there is no theory of EF.

All three of these problems pertain to a much larger fourth problem. That issue is contained in the question Why EF? (Barkley, 2001). This is a different question from those raised above. Without answering it one is likely to get only partial answers to the other questions. To answer why humans developed EF, one must think about ultimate ends. For what purposes does EF exist? What is it accomplishing? What problem(s) in human daily existence does this mental mechanism, or more likely suite of mental mechanisms, exist to solve? The only explanation for that question comes out of evolution. Thus, this book will take an evolutionary or "adaptationist" stance in addressing the question Why EF?

This book seeks to address all four of these issues. Each will now be discussed in more detail to support the contention that these *are* serious problems even if 160+ years of history has made it seem as if they had been resolved. If there is to be further advancement of our understanding of the concept of EF, these problems stand in our way.

What Is EF?: The Lack of an Operational Definition

Sidebar 1.1 lists a variety of definitions of EF. There is much cross-referencing among many of them, but this does not clarify or operationalize the term any better; it just sidesteps the problem and kicks the conceptual can further down the road. To illustrate the point, consider one of the most popular definitions appearing in the literature on EF, particularly in research on normal children and people having ADHD (Hinshaw, Carte, Fan, Jassy, & Owen, 2007; Martel, Nikolas, & Nigg, 2007; Rhodes, Coghill, & Matthews, 2005; Wilding, 2005; Willcutt, Doyle, Nigg, Faraone, & Pennington, 2005). While many of the authors citing this definition attribute it to Welsh and Pennington (1988), the latter authors credit it to Luria (1966). But Luria credits it to Bianchi (1895, 1922) as well as to the writings of Bekhterev (1905–1907). The definition states:

> Executive function is defined as the ability to maintain an appropriate problem-solving set for attainment of a future goal. (Welsh & Pennington, 1988, pp. 201–202)

Neither this definition nor any of those in Sidebar 1.1 indicate which mental function or tests of that mental function would be considered "executive" and which would not qualify for that distinction. Clearly this is not a single "ability." Welsh and Pennington (1988) went on to specify the components of EF as being

> a) an intention to inhibit a response or to defer it to a later more appropriate time; b) a strategic plan of action sequences; and c) a mental representation of the task, including the relevant stimulus information encoded in memory and the desired future goal-state. (p. 202)

SIDEBAR 1.1. A Sampling of Definitions of EF

The frontal cortex is critically involved in implementing executive progammes where these are necessary to maintain brain organization in the face of insufficient redundancy in input processing and in the outcomes of behavior. (Pribram, 1973, p. 301)

The executive functions consist of those capacities that enable a person to engage successfully in independent, purposive, self-serving behavior. They differ from cognitive functions in a number of ways. Questions about executive functions ask *how* and *whether* a person goes about doing something (e.g., Will you do it and if so, how?); questions about cognitive functions are generally phrased in terms of *what* or *how much* (e.g., How much do you know? What can you do?). (Lezak, 1995, p. 42)

The executive functions can be conceptualized as having four components: (1) volition; (2) planning; (3) purposive action; and (4) effective performance. Each involves a distinctive set of activity-related behaviors. All are necessary for appropriate, socially responsible, and effectively self-serving adult conduct. Moreover, it is rare to find a patient with impaired capacity for self-direction and self-regulation who has defects in just one of these aspects of executive functioning. Rather, defective executive behavior typically involves a cluster of deficiencies of which one or two may be especially prominent. (Lezak, 1995, p. 650)

The term "executive functioning" generally refers to the mechanisms by which performance is optimized in situations requiring the operation of a number of cognitive processes (Baddeley, 1986). Executive function is required when effective new plans of action must be formulated, and appropriate sequences of responses must be selected and scheduled. (Robbins, 1996, p. 1463). [Robbins goes on to identify working memory, inhibition, and monitoring of behavior relative to internal affective and motivational states as likely components of EF.]

[Executive functions are] a range of poorly defined processes which are putatively involved in activities such as "problem-solving," . . . "planning" . . . "initiation" of activity, "cognitive estimation," and "prospective memory." (Burgess, 1997, p. 81)

The executive functions are a collection of processes that are responsible for guiding, directing, and managing cognitive, emotional, and behavioral functions, particularly during active, novel problem solving. The term *executive function* represents an umbrella construct that includes a collection of inter-related functions that are responsible for purposeful, goal-directed, problem-solving behavior. (Gioia et al., 2000, p. 1)

(*continued*)

SIDEBAR 1.1. (*continued*)

Executive function (EF) is an umbrella term that incorporates a collection of inter-related processes responsible for purposeful, goal-directed behavior (Gioia, Isquith, & Guy, 2001). These executive processes are essential for the synthesis of external stimuli, formation of goals and strategies, preparation for action, and verification that plans and actions have been implemented appropriately (Luria, 1973). Processes associated with EF are numerous, but the principal elements include anticipation, goal selection, planning, initiation of activity, self-regulation, mental flexibility, deployment of attention, and utilization of feedback. (Anderson, 2002, p. 71)

Executive functions refer to a collection of interrelated cognitive and behavioral skills that are responsible for purposeful, goal-directed activity, and include the highest level of human functioning, such as intellect, thought, self-control, and social interaction (Lezak, 1995, p. 42). More specifically, executive functions are responsible for coordinating the activities involved in goal completion such as anticipation, goal selection, planning, initiation of activity, self-regulation, deployment of attention, and utilization of feedback. (Anderson et al., 2002, p. 231)

Executive functions is a generic term that refers to a variety of different capacities that enable purposeful, goal-directed behavior, including behavioral regulation, working memory, planning and organizational skills, and self-monitoring (Stuss & Benson, 1986). (Mangeot et al., 2002, p. 272)

EF encompasses metacognitive processes that enable efficient planning, execution, verification, and regulation of goal directed behavior. There is no single agreed upon definition of EF. (Oosterlaan, Scheres, & Sergeant, 2005, p. 69)

[Executive functioning is] an umbrella term for various cognitive processes that subserve goal-directed behavior (Miller & Cohen, 2001; Luria, 1966; Shallice, 1982). EF is especially important in novel or demanding situations (Stuss, 1992) which require a rapid and flexible adjustment of behavior to the changing demands of the environment (Zelazo, Muller, Frye, & Marcovitch, 2003). (Huizinga, Dolan, & van der Molen, 2006, p. 217)

Executive functions have been notoriously difficult to define precisely. For example, Sergeant, Geurts, & Oosterlaan (2002) note that there are "33 definitions of EF" (p. 3). However, most investigators would agree that EFs are self-regulatory functions incorporating the ability to inhibit, shift set, organize, use working memory, problem solve, and maintain set for future goals (Pennington & Ozonoff, 1996; Sergeant et al., 2002). (Seidman et al., 2006, p. 166)

[Executive functions comprise] a family of cognitive control processes that operate on lower-level processes to regulate and shape behavior. (Friedman et al., 2007, p. 893)

The umbrella concept of "executive control" encompasses those cognitive functions involved in the selection, scheduling and coordination of the computational processes responsible for perception, memory and action (Norman & Shallice, 1986; Shallice, 1994). [EF enables] the maintenance of behavior on a goal set and calibration of behavior to context (Pennington & Ozonoff, 1996). (Ciairano, Visu-Petra, & Settanni, 2007, p. 335)

EF involves developing and implementing an approach to performing a task that is not habitually performed (Mahone et al., 2002). The early development of skills that support EF includes the ability to maintain problem-solving set for attainment of future goal (Welsh & Pennington, 1988), and encompasses an individual's ability to inhibit actions, restrain and delay responses, attend selectivity [sic], self-regulate, problem solve, be flexible, set goals, plan, and shift set (Senn, Espy, & Kaufmann, 2004; Singer & Bashir, 1999). (Mahone & Hoffman, 2007, pp. 569–570)

Executive functioning has been defined as a set of regulatory processes necessary for selecting, initiating, implementing, and overseeing thought, emotion, behavior, and certain facets of motor and sensory functions (Roth, Isquith, & Gioia, 2005). (Schroeder & Kelley, 2009, pp. 227–228)

In general, executive function can be thought of as the set of abilities required to effortfully guide behavior toward a goal, especially in nonroutine situations. Various functions are thought to fall under the rubric of executive function. These include prioritizing and sequencing behavior, inhibiting familiar and stereotyped behaviors, creating and maintaining an idea of what task or information is most relevant for current purposes (often referred to as an attentional or mental set), providing resistance to information that is distracting or task irrelevant, switching behavior task goals, utilizing relevant information in support of decision making, categorizing or otherwise abstracting common elements across items, and handling novel information or situations. As can be seen from this list, the functions that fall under the category of executive function are indeed wide ranging. (Banich, 2009, p. 89)

EF includes processing related to goal-directed behavior, or the control of complex cognition, especially in nonroutine situations (Banich, 2009; Fuster, 1997; Lezak, 1995). (McCabe, Roediger, McDaniel, Balota, & Hambrick, 2010, p. 222)

But why is only this set of three mental abilities included in EF and not others? Why is maintaining an appropriate problem-solving set toward a future goal considered to be the essential nature of EF? Wouldn't it be more precise and simpler to just make these three components part of the definition of EF itself? For instance, EF is the inhibition of a response or its deferral to a more appropriate time so as to develop a mental representation of the task and desired future goal, develop a strategic plan of action sequences to attain it, and maintain an appropriate problem-solving set toward that future goal.

For instance, why is it that detecting and responding to an X on a computer screen while inhibiting a response to an O is an executive function test, while reading an X when it appears is not? Or why is stating the color of ink in which a color word (i.e., "red") is printed considered an executive function but reading the actual printed word is not? Or why is pointing to a location where a picture or geometric design appeared in a matrix after it has disappeared for a few seconds an indication of EF, while pointing to the same design in the matrix while it is still present is not an EF? Why is sorting cards into categories based on your own sorting rule not an EF, while sorting them so as to discover an examiner's undisclosed sorting rule is considered an EF? Such distinctions cry out for an operational definition of the term "EF," yet none that is currently available can manage even these distinctions.

To muddy these waters even further, consider the fact that Eslinger (1996) described a conference (which I attended) held in January 1994 at the National Institute of Child Health and Human Development (Washington, D.C.) in which 10 experts in EF were asked to generate terms that would be considered executive functions. They came up with 33! The greatest agreement (endorsed by 40% or more of the participants) existed for the following six components of EF: self-regulation, sequencing of behavior, flexibility, response inhibition, planning, and organization of behavior. Why these? Using a consensus of opinion is akin to conducting science by democratic vote, fashion, or mob rule; it does nothing to advance the clarity or operationalizing of a definition of a scientific construct such as EF. As another example of the dog's breakfast of constructs that EF has become, Best, Miller, and Jones (2009) reviewed the evidence on the development of EF and identified at least 15 components in contemporary research. Among these, Best et al. (2009) settled on the most important four for their review based largely on the frequency with which they had appeared in earlier research. They argued that these components likely develop at different rates and probably in the following sequence: (1) inhibition, (2) working memory, (3) shifting, and (4) planning (which includes problem solving). Why just classify these four as EF out of the 15 identified in the review? The fact that measures of these four constructs often outnumbered those of others in the research under review does not necessarily make them important for understanding EF; it is only an indication of a psychometric popularity contest.

Again, however, one can rightly ask why these constructs of response inhibition, working memory, planning, and flexibility or set shifting are often classified as EF but visual–spatial perception, speech and language, emotion, and motor speed and coordination, among others, are not (Lyon & Krasnegor, 1996; Stuss & Benson, 1986)? Surely one can argue that the latter mental abilities help to maintain problem solving for attainment of a goal. If you cannot locate your position in space, there are many goals you are not going to be able to pursue. What is the essential nature of EF that renders the former within its domain but excludes the latter? Given such a polyglot of constructs incorporated under the EF tent, it is no wonder that the field has made little headway in its development of useful operational definitions of EF in the past 30 years. Apart from the fact that many of these EF components can be largely (though not entirely) localized to various regions of the PFC, just what makes these mental capacities or modules an EF at the neuropsychological level of definition and analysis? Are we to be stuck with mere reductionism to the neuroanatomical level as the only means of defining what constitutes EF?

How Is EF Assessed?: The Poor Ecological Validity of Psychometric Tests of EF

The second problem this book intends to address is rooted in the first problem—absent an operational definition of EF, what methods will qualify as measures of it? The field of neuropsychology seems to have answered this question by largely focusing on the use of psychometric tests as the principal or sole basis for evaluating EF deficits in clinical patients and in research studies. Indeed, it seems that the field of neuropsychology is synonymous with psychometrics. Other than convenience or tradition, why are tests given in clinical or lab settings the widespread basis for measuring EF, and not direct observations of human action in natural settings or rating scales completed by patients and others? Over the past 40 years occasional voices have been raised warning that neuropsychological tests of EF were problematic. The tests were unlikely to be capturing much of what is considered to be the essence of EF or its important features as humans use it in their daily life or to be adversely affected by injuries to the PFC (Barkley, 2001; Dimond, 1980; Dodrill, 1997; Lezak, 2004; Rabbitt, 1997; Shallice & Burgess, 1991). The warnings have largely gone unheeded as EF tests and test batteries have come to represent an inchoate gold standard for determining EF and its deficits. With very few exceptions, the vast majority of studies published on the topic of EF have used EF tests or batteries of tests to determine whether certain disorders impaired EF or how EF developed in normal samples.

This would be fine if these tests were highly reliable and well validated. But they are not. Research consistently shows such tests to be of only moderate or lower reliability (Lezak, 2004; Rabbitt, 1997). They are also of limited utility for detecting PFC injuries (Dodrill, 1997). For example, only a minority of patients experiencing frontal lobe injuries or those with ADHD known to have a frontal lobe disorder score in the impaired range on these measures. In contrast, consider the fact that the vast majority of such patients place in that range of impairment on ratings of EF in daily life activities or in direct observations of EF performance in natural settings (Alderman, Burgess, Knight, & Henman, 2003; Barkley & Murphy, 2010; Burgess, Alderman, Evans, Emslie, & Wilson, 1998; Gioia, Isquith, Kenworthy, & Barton, 2002; Kertesz, Nadkarni, Davidson, & Thomas, 2000; Mitchell & Miller, 2008; Wood & Liossi, 2006). This tells us that people with PFC disorders and injuries have EF deficits in their daily life activities even if the EF tests do not detect them. And it is the deficits occurring in daily life, not those manifested on tests, that are the most important to understand and to clinically assess and rehabilitate or manage.

This leads to the second problem with EF tests. They have little or no ecological validity. In other words, these tests do not correlate well, if at all, with more ecologically valid means of assessing EF in everyday life circumstances. This has been evident repeatedly in studies of these tests in comparison to systematic observations, structured interviews, or ratings of daily self-care and adaptive functioning, and to behavior ratings of EF in adults (Alderman et al., 2003; Bogod, Mateer, & MacDonald, 2003; Burgess et al., 1998; Chaytor, Schmitter-Edgecombe, & Burr, 2006; Mitchell & Miller, 2008; Ready, Stierman, & Paulsen, 2001; Wood & Liossi, 2006). The same problem is evident in children with frontal lobe lesions, traumatic brain injuries (TBI), or other neurological or developmental disorders (Anderson, Anderson, Northam, Jacobs, & Mikiewicz, 2002; Mangeot, Armstrong, Colvin, Yeates, & Taylor, 2002; Vriezen & Pigott, 2002; Zandt, Prior, & Kirios, 2009). This is also the case in both adults with ADHD and children with ADHD followed to adulthood (Barkley & Fischer, 2011; Barkley & Murphy, 2011). If a primary clinical aim is to predict how well an individual will do with executive functioning in the real world of their daily life activities, then EF tests are of minimal or no help.

The results of these various studies usually reveal that any single EF test shares just 0–10% of its variance with EF ratings or observations of

EF in daily adaptive functioning. The relationships are frequently not statistically significant. Even the best combination of EF tests shares just 9–20% of the variance with EF ratings or observations as reflected in these studies (Barkley & Fischer, 2011; Barkley & Murphy, 2011; O'Shea et al., 2010; Ready et al., 2001; Stavro, Ettenhofer, & Nigg, 2007; Zandt et al., 2009). If IQ is statistically removed from the results, the few significant relationships found in these studies between EF tests and EF ratings may even become nonsignificant (Mangeot et al., 2002). Yet these two methods are supposed to be measuring the same construct—EF. In contrast, research has noted moderate relationships between EF ratings and measures of daily adaptive functioning in children with various disorders including TBI (Gilotty, Kenworthy, Sirian, Black, & Wagner, 2002; Mangeot et al., 2002), in adults with ADHD (Barkley & Murphy, 2011; Biederman et al., 2007), in children with ADHD followed to adulthood (Barkley & Fischer, 2011), in people with frontal lobe disorders (Alderman et al., 2003), in college undergraduates (Ready et al., 2001), or in other populations (O'Shea et al., 2010). Something is terribly amiss here if different methods of measuring the same construct are so poorly related to each other and lead to such disparate findings and hence conclusions.

There is also the problem with the low and often nonsignificant predictive validity of EF tests. If EF is such an important, if not *the* most important, mental faculty of humans, as some have argued (Luria, 1966; Stuss & Benson, 1986), then tests of EF or its deficits should be significantly predictive of impairments in various major life activities such as occupational functioning, educational history, driving, money management, and criminal conduct. But they are not or are very poor at doing so (Barkley & Fischer, 2011; Barkley & Murphy, 2010, 2011).

The totality of findings to date concerning the relationship of EF tests to EF ratings and of each to impairment in daily life indicates that EF tests are largely not sampling the same constructs as are EF ratings or direct evaluations of EF in daily life (Alderman et al., 2003; Shallice & Burgess, 1991). It also provides a basis for not accepting EF tests as the primary or sole source for establishing the nature of EF deficits in various disorders or of its development in studies of normal samples. In sum, EF tests should not serve as the gold standard for evaluating EF.

This significant failure of EF tests to relate well to EF ratings, daily life activities, or impairment in major domains of life could well indicate that the tests are not assessing EF. This seems arguable given that many of these tests have been shown to index activities in various regions of the PFC that largely underlie EF. But it is surely unlikely to be the case that EF ratings are not actually evaluating EF. After all, their item content has been drafted directly from various descriptions of EF and from lists of putative EF constructs in the literature as well as from observations and clinical descriptions of patients with PFC lesions believed to manifest the "dysexecutive syndrome" (Barkley, 2011a; Burgess et al., 1998; Gioia, Iquith, Guy, & Kenworthy, 2000; Kertesz et al., 2000). Moreover, as noted above, these ratings are substantially related to impairment in various daily life activities and various domains of adaptive functioning, such as work, education, driving, social relationships, and self-sufficiency, in which EF would surely be operative.

Adding insult to injury in this field of research, the nearly slavish devotion to the use of EF tests as the sole or gold standard for its evaluation has resulted in some serious logical errors in various research studies on EF and reviews of that literature. For instance, my own area of clinical and research specialization is ADHD. The following current situation in this field represents this error:

- The PFC is the "executive" brain (Pribram, 1973).
- ADHD is a disorder arising largely from structural and functional abnormalities in the PFC (Bush, Valera, & Seidman, 2005; Valera, Faraone, Murray, & Seidman, 2007).
- ADHD is largely *not* a disorder of EF (Boonstra, Oosterlaan, Sergeant, & Buitelaar, 2005; Jonsdottir, Bouma, Sergeant, & Scherder, 2006; Marchetta, Hurks, Krabbendam, & Jolles, 2008; Nigg, Wilcutt, Doyle, & Sonuga-Barke, 2005; Willcutt et al., 2005).

The last conclusion was reached because the studies cited above and others (Barkley & Fischer, 2011; Barkley & Murphy, 2011; Biederman et al., 2008) demonstrated that the majority of individuals with ADHD are not impaired on EF tests, even if groups of ADHD cases differ in mean scores from control groups on many such tests (Frazier, Demareem, & Youngstrom, 2004; Hervey, Epstein, & Curry, 2004). So if EF tests are to be the sole standard for assessing the presence of EF deficits, then most cases of ADHD do not have such deficits. Ergo, ADHD is not a disorder of EF in most cases. This logical error has been repeated countless times with other disorders. For instance, a recent study concluded that the risk for developing a substance use disorder in adolescence or young adulthood is unrelated to the presence of EF deficits in childhood or adolescence—a conclusion reached solely on the basis of EF tests (Wilens et al., 2011). Such studies of disorders and the role of EF in them that relied exclusively on the psychometric approach to evaluating EF obviously now have their conclusions greatly restricted by the qualifier "as measured by EF tests." The same caveat applies as well to studies of the normal course of development of EF. These studies will need to be redone using other approaches to evaluate EF before any conclusions about EF involvement in these disorders or normal processes have any validity and generality and so can be taken seriously.

In short, why are putative EF tests so insensitive to injuries of the executive brain—the PFC? Why are they so poorly related to EF ratings and direct observations of EF-related activities in daily human life? And why are these tests so much worse at predicting impairment in adaptive functioning and major life activities than are the EF ratings? A second aim of this book is to bridge this gap between these psychometric versus ethological methods of assessing EF to show how this state of affairs could arise, what it means for conceptualizing EF, and how to resolve it.

How Does EF Work?: The Limitations of Current Cognitive Models of EF

The third problem that arises and contributes to the first two above lies in how EF works. As noted earlier, we can conceptualize EF as a construct or set of constructs. But to know how it works we must propose relationships among constructs and explain how they operate—we must have a theory. The functions of the PFC, or the executive brain, have been the subject of medical and scientific scrutiny for more than 160 years. Initial efforts to elucidate these functions relied largely on the study of the symptoms and deficits evident in individuals who had suffered serious injuries to this region of the brain. Among the first and most famous of such cases was that of Phineas Gage, the railroad foreman who suffered a penetrating head wound that destroyed a large portion of his PFC. This led to drastic alterations in his behavior, personality, and social conduct (Harlow, 1848, 1868). Like Gage, patients with PFC damage studied in these early years demonstrated a lack of initiative or drive, a curtailing of their circle of interests, profound disturbances of goal-directed behavior, a loss of abstract or categorical behavior, and emotional changes, such as a proneness to irritation, emotional instability, and indifference toward their surroundings, often superimposed on depression (Fuster, 1997; Luria, 1966; Stuss & Benson, 1986). Impulsive actions, trivial jokes, and even euphoria were noted to arise from lesions that involved the more basal aspects of the PFC. Just as likely was an adverse impact on moral conduct, independence and self-reliance, financial-economic self-support, effective occupational performance, and socially cooperative activities that all require the capacity for evaluating the longer-term consequences of one's actions as noted in the initial report on Gage (Harlow, 1848).

Luria (1966) gives a fine account of the subsequent history of the study of the functions of the frontal lobes. From him we learn that Hughlings Jackson is said to have viewed the PFC as "the highest motor centres" being "the most complex and least organized centres" (Luria, 1966, p. 221). According to Luria (1966), Bianchi (1895) voiced similar views independently of Jackson, arguing that the frontal lobes contained the most complex forms of reflex activity organized hierarchically into a series of levels that "bring about the widest coordination of sensory and motor elements, utilize the product of the sensory zones to create mental syntheses, and play the same role in relation to the sensorimotor (or kinesthetic) zones that the latter play in relation to the subcortical nuclei" (Luria, 1966, p. 221). This was the integrative function first attributed to the prefrontal lobes. Both Bekhterev (1905–1907) and later Pavlov (see Luria, 1966, p. 222) observed that damaging the prefrontal lobes resulted in a disintegration of goal-directed behavior, which they saw as the principal function of the PFC. This later became the basis for the Welsh and Pennington (1988) definition of EF, as noted above.

Additional subsequent research noted other deficits evident in individuals with damage to the PFC. These included being "easily distracted by extraneous stimuli" (Luria, 1966, p. 224) including extraneous thoughts or patterns of irrelevant mental associations (Luria, 1966, p. 286), and being unable to develop or sustain a readiness for action or intentional quality to their actions. Patients were frequently noted to be hyperactive as a consequence of the poor inhibition of the lower, more automatic forms of behavior. Studies of animals whose PFC had been intentionally ablated manifested similar symptoms and deficits. Hence the integration and execution of goal-directed behavior, the inhibition of more automatic actions and reactions to extraneous stimuli (distractibility), the production of delayed reactions, the evaluation of one's goal-directed actions relative to the external environment, especially in novel circumstances, and the overall intentionality or purposive quality of behavior were all functions attributable to the PFC.

Luria goes on to state that "besides the disturbance of initiative and the other aforementioned behavioral disturbances, almost all patients with a lesion of the frontal lobes have a marked loss of their 'critical faculty,' i.e., a disturbance of their ability to correctly evaluate their own behavior and the adequacy of their actions" (1966, p. 227). Impaired here was a faculty of relational comparisons between the patients' goals, their current actions relative to those goals, their actions relative to others while in pursuit of those goals, and the environmental feedback as to the effectiveness of those actions vis-à-vis the goal. This is similar to the observations of Freeman and Watts (1941) that the frontal lobes are concerned with self-awareness, that is, with foresight and the relation of the self (current) to the self (future). PFC-injured patients also demonstrated a marked impairment in voluntary movement and activity. Such movements are unique to humans. They are a response to either verbal instruction from others or the formation of an intention of their own translated into a self-instruction. Today, these would be considered forms of rule-governed behavior (Hayes, 1989; Hayes, Gifford, & Ruckstuhl, 1996) or what Luria called the regulating functions of speech (1966, p. 250).

Damage to the PFC was typically accompanied by a release of more automatic forms of behavior. For instance, this might be seen in the inappropriate utilization of an object for its intended purposes in the wrong context as described by Lhermitte, Pillon, and Serdaru (1986). It would also be manifest in the perseveration of actions, despite a change in the context that should have led to a termination of those actions, and in impulsive responses to irrelevant events (Luria, 1966). The totality of this pattern of deficits came to be known as a frontal lobe syndrome. Later, when Pribram (1973, 1976) referred to the functions of the PFC as "executive" in nature, this would subsequently lead to the frontal lobe syndrome being known as a "dysexecutive syndrome" (Wilson, Alderman, Burgess, Emslie, & Evans, 1996).

Some contemporary theories of EF are briefly summarized in Sidebar 1.2. My intent here is not to comprehensively review such models or discuss each in detail. But such theories are all fraught to varying degrees with a set of problems. Briefly elucidating those problems will suffice to show that further theory-building about EF is in order.

The Disparity between Models of EF and Deficits in Patients with PFC Disorders

Recall the array of cognitive, behavioral, emotional, social, economic, and moral impairments associated with damage to the human executive brain discussed above and as evident in any neurology or neuropsychology clinic that specializes in their care. Now contrast them with contem-

SIDEBAR 1.2. A Sampling of Theories of PFC (EF) Functioning

Stuss and Benson's Hierarchical Model of EF

A commonly cited early conceptualization of EF was that specified by Stuss and Benson (1986) in their book on the frontal lobes:

> Executive control functions, called into action in nonroutine or novel situations, provide conscious direction to the functional systems for efficient processing of information. . . . The executive function represents many of the important activities that are almost universally attributed to the frontal lobes which become active in nonroutine, novel situations that require new solutions. These behavioral characteristics have been described by many authors and include at least the following: anticipation, goal selection, preplanning (means-end establishment), monitoring, and use of feedback (if–then statements). (p. 244)

In this model, EF refers to four components (anticipation, goal selection, preplanning, and monitoring). In their diagram of PFC functions, Stuss and Benson place these EF components above two other frontal modules that they are said to govern: Drive (drive, motivation, and will) and Sequencing (sequence, set, and integration). In this model, drive and sequencing are not EF. Drive, motivation, and will comprise the first (Drive) of the two modules governed by the EF control system (p. 243). In it, drive refers to basic appetitive states that are basic energizing forces. Motivation is conceived as being more mental/intellectual control of drive states. And "will" is undefined but is implied to be an even higher state that governs motivation, most likely representing consciously conceived wants or desires.

The second of these modules (Sequencing) is said to be involved in organizing and maintaining bits of information into meaningful sequences, such as in the temporal integration and sequencing of behavior. Stuss and Benson cite Fuster's work in support of the existence of this module (see Fuster, 1997). Fuster argued that three subordinate functions are needed to organize and integrate behavior across time: anticipation (the prospective function), provisional memory (working memory), and control of interference (the inhibitory function). To these functions, Stuss and Benson added the synthetic capacity to form sets of related information that allows the production of new, more complex information from available sequences of data. With this also goes the capacity for the integration of a number of related and unrelated sets of information into novel knowledge and hence novel action (see pp. 241–242).

These two modules (Drive, Sequencing) govern the nonexecutive posterior/basal functional systems, such as attention, alertness, visual–spatial, autonomic emotional, memory, sensory/perception, language, motor, and cognition. Interestingly, perched above the EF level and atop all of these components is Self-Awareness, believed to be the highest attribute of the frontal lobes (see Figure 17.4 in Stuss & Benson, 1986). It is viewed as separable from EF and is hierarchically placed above it (pp. 246–247). Noteworthy from this perspective is that self-awareness is implied, if not declared, to be the central executive that determines the activities of the lower level functions, including the EF level.

Fuster's Theory of Cross-Temporal Organization

A widely cited theory of PFC functioning that similarly deals with goal-directed behavior is Fuster's (1997) model of cross-temporal synthesis or integration. Cross-temporal synthesis is based on three PFC components: (1) working memory, which is a temporally retrospective function; (2) anticipatory set (planning), which is a temporally prospective function; and (3) interference control (a form of attention that involves resistance to distraction), which inhibits the disruption of goal-directed behavior by events or behavior that are irrelevant to or incompatible with the goal. Fuster argues that the overarching purpose of these three EF components is "the cross-temporal organization of behavior" (1997, p. 157). This is achieved by a *temporal synthesis* or integration that represents the "formation of *temporal structures of behavior* with a unifying purpose or goal—in other words, the structuring of goal-directed behavior" (p. 158). Like Stuss and Benson (1986), Fuster includes in his concept of EF the self-regulation of motivational, emotional, and other drive states in the service of goal-directed behavior.

Central to this model of PFC/EF is the need to appreciate that goal-directed actions often involve significant delays among events (E), responses (R), and goals and their attendant consequences (G/C). Such lengthy delays require an internal means of temporal structuring or binding together the components of this contingency. This, Fuster argues, is done by mentally representing the E-R-G/C arrangement. Goal-directed behavior is achieved through the guidance of behavior by these internal representations, and those representations arise from his three components. To Fuster, EF "is closely related, if not identical, to the function of temporal synthesis of action, which rests on the same subordinate functions. Temporal synthesis, however, does not need a central executive" (p. 165). Fuster does not put a ghost in the machine or homunculus in the mind. All along, it is the individual organism that is selecting what goals it will pursue within the constraints of its time horizon or capacity for retrospective and prospective functions.

While Fuster acknowledges that PFC-injured patients display an inordinate degree of concreteness in their daily behavior, he believes that this is largely, if not solely, a temporal concreteness. "The patient suffers from an overall constriction of the scope and complexity of behavior and of the thinking behind it" (p. 165). Behavioral patterns that are not well established are anchored in the present, devoid of temporal perspective, for the past as well as the future, and have an air of temporal immediacy dominated by immediate needs and stimuli or the here and now. In this model, once a desire, want, or goal comes into mind, the temporal integration or synthesis activities of the frontal lobes serve to construct the cross-temporal chains of behavior necessary to its attainment and, if thwarted, the problem-solving mental manipulations that may be needed to surmount the obstacle. Deficits in any of the three can result

(continued)

SIDEBAR 1.2. (*continued*)

in deficient temporal integration of behavior, or EF, and thus lead to different forms or origins of EF deficits. EF (temporal synthesis) depends on all three of Fuster's components, and hence deficits in any component give rise to a distinct disorder of EF.

Duncan's Theory of Goal Neglect

A less complex theory of the functions of the PFC is that of goal neglect by Duncan (1986). It essentially argues that human behavior is organized around a list of goals and subgoals against which individuals are comparing their ongoing behavior to maintain behavior directed at these goals. Frontal lobe damage results in an inability to retain these goals in mind and thus greater disorganization of behavior.

Borkowski and Burke's Information-Processing Theory of EF

Most of the definitions or descriptions of the PFC's functions given above arose out of clinical observations of patients with frontal lobe injuries or ablation studies of animals. An alternative perspective to EF developed in the 1990s out of information-processing theory. Typical of this was the work of Borkowski and Burke (1996) and other authors whose work they summarized in this field. Borkowski and Burke described EF as a set of three components that are directed at problem solving: task analysis (essentially defining the problem), strategy selection and revision, and strategy monitoring. Those authors also cited a different information-processing model developed by Butterfield and Albertson (1995) that views executive functioning as one of three components of cognition: cognition, metacognition, and executive functioning.

> Cognition is all the knowledge and strategies that exist in long-term memory; this reservoir of information is critical to effective problem solving. The metacognitive level is aware of this lower level and contains models of the various cognitive processes as well as an understanding of how knowledge and strategies interconnect. Executive functioning coordinates these two levels of cognition by monitoring and controlling the use of the knowledge and strategies in concordance with the metacognitive level. (Borkowski & Burke, 1996, p. 241)

Another model from cognitive psychology acknowledged by Borkowski and Burke (1996) in their review was that of Bransford and Stein (1993) and their model of the IDEAL problem solver that included EF in that model. IDEAL is the acronym for the components of the model: (1) *i*dentify an important problem to be solved, (2) *d*efine the subgoals involved in solving the problem, (3) *e*xplore the possible approaches to the problem (select a potential set of strategies), (4) *a*nticipate potential outcomes before acting on the best initial approach, and (5) *l*ook back and learn from the entire problem-solving experience. If problem solving is to be a component of EF, then this usefully makes explicit what steps are being used in that component. The steps here overlap with the Borkowski and Burke model and that of Butterfield and Albertson above. These steps are also highly similar to Scholnick and Friedman's (1993) model of *planning*. Hence planning and problem solving may be synonymous terms, although planning seems to also include a longer-term future consideration than might problem solving, which can be applied to much more near-term problems. Still, both models include a component of problem selection (choosing an important problem implies a futuristic feature perhaps) and certainly anticipation of outcomes that include some time horizon over which problems/goals and actions are to be considered.

Borkowski and Burke (1996) admit that self-regulation, planning, and EF overlap but argue that they have some distinctions. Planning, they claim, necessitates decision making, regulation, and action. They view self-regulation as a component of planning but limited to the strategies necessary to achieve desired goal states. EF, like self-regulation, is a component of planning because planning has more generality in its application, whereas EF may be less so. In their view EF only involves task analysis and related steps (strategy selection/ revision, self-monitoring). These may be distinctions without a difference, or variations on a common theme of goal-directed action. Surprisingly, Borkowski and Burke (1996) do not include inhibition in their EF model and yet admit that deficiencies in it would spill over into their components of EF and be detrimental to them.

Hayes's Behavioral Theory of EF as Rule-Governed Behavior

A quite different view of EF was proposed at this same time by Hayes et al. (1996) using a more behavioral analytic model, particularly the concept of rule-governed behavior (see Hayes, 1989). Their analysis of the terms often believed to comprise EF as well as many of the tests used to assess EF led them to conclude that EF is a special subset of rule-governed (verbally regulated) behavior. Rule-governed behavior is behavior that is being initiated and guided by verbalizations, whether self-directed or provided by others. We saw elements of the importance of this type of PFC function in the work of Luria (1966) above.

Hayes et al. argued that EF tasks place people in situations where previously learned sources of behavioral regulation come into conflict with rules laid down by the task and examiner. Those task-specific rules are competing with behavior that is otherwise automatic and well practiced. Thus, the typical automatic flow of behavior must be interrupted and delayed long enough for the person to discover a new rule or select among previously learned rules that may apply in this situation. Yet interrupting a well-practiced behavior itself often requires that a rule be selected and followed that is initiating the delay in responding. And so in EF tasks individuals often have to implement a rule to inhibit their usual ongoing responding, even if it is just asking them a question about the task. They must then either select from among a set of relevant previously learned rules or generate a new one. The latter is a verbal means

(continued)

SIDEBAR 1.2. (*continued*)

by which we problem solve, as in the five steps to problem solving discussed above, which are second order rules used to discover first-order rules.

Discovering or selecting the rule is only part of the process, for the individual must now follow it, adhere to it, or "track" the rule. Pliance may occur, where immediate and artificial consequences are applied to motivate the rule following, or tracking may occur where the natural consequences have now taken over to sustain the behavior. Sometimes augmenting is also needed where verbal self-reinforcement (or statements by others) is also used for motivation, as in phrases such as "good boy," or self-statements of being right or being good in following the rule. This view of EF appeared to gain little favor among traditional neuropsychologists who seemed more comfortable using a cognitive neuropsychological or information-processing view of EF than one derived from behavior analysis. Yet features of it would be incorporated into my own model of EF (Barkley, 1997a, 1997b) through Vygotsky's model of the internalization of self-directed speech (1987).

---

porary definitions of EF, as shown in Sidebar 1.1, and even against several contemporary models of EF as shown in Sidebar 1.2. These contemporary views of EF rarely, if ever, refer to emotional, social, economic, occupational, or moral deficits associated with these earlier descriptions of PFC injuries or EF deficits. What one observes instead is a near exclusive focus on the rather narrower "cold" cognitive constructs that are now thought to be included within the term "EF," such as response inhibition, working memory, set shifting, sustained attention, planning and problem solving, and fluency or generativity (Castellanos, Sonuga-Barke, Milham, & Tannock, 2006; Nigg & Casey, 2005; Nigg & Casey, 2005). As noted earlier, up to 33 such constructs have been placed under the umbrella of EF in modern views of this concept. So variously defined is EF that some authors simply skip defining EF entirely (Biederman et al., 2008; Gilotty et al., 2002; Papadopoulos, Panayiotou, Spanoudis, & Natsopoulos, 2005), proceeding instead to directly listing one or a few constructs they believe to represent EF, such as response inhibition (Hale et al., 2009), and working memory, set shifting, and planning (Castellanos et al., 2006; Willcutt et al., 2005).

From these constructs, as noted above, psychometric tests are then selected for use as EF tests or test batteries, and the results of the studies are said to reflect the extent to which certain clinical disorders involve EF or to which EF may develop in normal samples. The result in my opinion has been a growing disconnection between contemporary cold cognitive research on EF and the widespread and often devastating behavioral, social, emotional, economic, occupational, and moral deficits so evident in the earlier descriptions of patients with PFC injuries or disorders. For example, how are we to see any connection between how patients perform a digit span backward, N-back, serial addition, or other task of verbal working memory and their economic life in their natural settings? Humans daily engage in reciprocal exchange and must frequently and rapidly evaluate the costs-benefits to them of doing so as each party to the transaction goes about pursuing their actions toward their future goals, no matter whether the exchange involves money, goods, or services. This is the field of economics, broadly defined. Yet where does this widespread human goal-directed activity ever enter into modern views of EF?

Consider how we are to connect the inability of PFC patients to sort cards into categories or reorganize rings onto spindles to match a sample arrangement and that individual's profound difficulties with ethical or moral conduct. What do such tasks tell us about the likelihood of the person having substantial difficulties with social relationships with others, with reciprocity and cooperation, or with participating in the community and obeying its laws? The fundamental basis of morality is awareness of one's self over time in relation to others and the future consequences of one's actions toward others and of others' toward one's self. This daily intersection of each human's goal-directed activities among those of other goal-directed humans requires rules (ethics) for making such activities run as smoothly and peaceably as possible. Where is this reflected in psychometric tests or modern cognitive models of EF? Such a myopic emphasis on short-term (minutes) cold cognitive psychometric tasks preferred by most contemporary neuropsychological studies has left a gapping chasm between the constructs sampled by these tests and the executive deficits evident in patients in their everyday life. This is the most likely reason why little or no relationship has been found between the tests and the observations and ratings of EF, adaptive functioning, and human major life activities saturated with EF, as discussed above.

When such cold cognitive models and tests based on them are then relied on to identify the dimensions or components of EF, further difficulties for theory-building can arise. Those cognitive tests further impede efforts to bridge the growing chasm between the results of modern studies into EF and the more widespread and socially devastating symptoms associated with PFC injuries and other EF disorders. Largely eschewing an attempt to operationally define the concept of EF, many authors have pursued a more empirical, atheoretical, statistical approach to understanding EF. This effort has chiefly been exemplified by attempts to factor analyze various batteries of putative EF tests to discover their underlying dimensions. Numerous such attempts have been made, with most identifying several distinct EF dimensions or factors. For instance, Miyake and colleagues (Miyake et al., 2000) used confirmatory factor analysis to determine whether the three most commonly proposed EF did, in fact, form distinct functions—these being set shifting, information updating, and inhibition. Using three tasks commonly used to assess these constructs and college students as participants, Miyake et al. found evidence for such a fractionating of EF. But Shute and Huertas (1990) also gave a battery of seven EF tasks to college students and identified four factors—flexibility/perseveration (or set shifting), perceptual–motor speed (probably not an EF), verbal working memory, and time estimation. These factors mainly reflected the tests in the battery. In Levin and colleagues' study of brain-injured children (Levin et al., 1996), five factors were identified from their battery of six EF tasks. Grodzinsky and Diamond (1992) gave a battery of 10 EF tests to their participants and found at least seven separate factors, most of which reflected the tests. Mariani and Barkley (1997) also used an extensive battery of EF and non-EF tests and identified at least four factors. Anderson (2002) described the results of several factor analyses of EF test batteries and the common factors they identified. These were planning, impulse control, and concept reasoning. A response speed factor was also found, but this would be considered nonexecutive. Anderson then goes on to develop his own four-factor model of EF: (1) attentional control (includes inhibition); (2) information processing (fluency, efficiency, and speed of output); (3) cognitive flexibility (shift response sets, learn from mistakes, devise alternative strategies, divide attention, process multiple sources of information concurrently); and (4) goal setting (develop new initiatives and concepts, plan actions in advance, approach tasks in an efficient and strategic manner).

But all of these findings could just as easily reflect method variance. As a general rule, the more tests included in the EF battery, the more factors the study seems to identify—these factors primarily comprise the different tests. It is therefore not clear that EF is as fractionated a construct as such studies suggest; nothing requires that it be conceptualized as such. What these studies more likely illustrate is that a diversity of putative tests of EF, when factor analyzed, result in a diversity of dimensions—as diverse as the tests included in the battery. Also troubling in this empirical (statistical) approach is that typically the correlations among these various factors are relatively and disturbingly low, suggesting only 10–20% of shared variance among them. This finding is not encouraging of a central construct or general EF factor (Lehto, 1996).

As Miyake and colleagues noted (Miyake et al., 2000), however, this limited relationship among the factors could just as easily reflect the diversity of non-EF abilities that are also being sampled in the EF test batteries. These non-EF abilities would obscure the commonality that might exist among them that would represent the higher order central executive faculty lying latent across these diverse tasks. Nevertheless, this sampling of research serves to illustrate the problem. The increased reliance on the psychometric approach to EF has resulted in relatively circumscribed cognitive faculties being incorporated into the term while failing to address the significant personal, emotional, social, economic, and moral deficits that frequently arise in disorders of the EF system—the PFC.

The Missing Linkage between EF and Social Functioning

Dimond (1980) and later Lezak (1995) were correct, I believe, in noting the relatively sparse recognition in the modern views of EF of its importance for social functioning and effectiveness, or what Dimond called our *social intelligence*. A few EF researchers have noted its importance, however, such as Ciairano and associates (Ciairano, Visu-Petra, & Settanni, 2007) on the importance of EF in cooperative social behavior. Dimond referred to "the capacity to respond to appropriate social patterns, to regulate social life and to integrate adequately and successfully with others" as being so important in PFC functioning (1980, p. 510).

> As one of its major functions, the frontal lobe bears responsibility for administering the code by which the patterns of social behavior are put into operation and by which the individual integrates and regulates its conduct in respect of that of other individuals. We postulated that there is a special form of social intelligence by which the organism maintains the running, changing stream of social relationships and that the frontal lobes bear important, if not unique, responsibility for this. (Dimond, 1980, p. 507)

There is a striking social pathology associated with PFC damage, Dimond (1980) argued, that goes largely unappreciated in efforts to describe the major functions of the PFC. Perhaps this is largely because clinicians and neuroscientists nearly always study such patients in isolation (individually) and in relatively short periods of time (a few hours at most at a time) in unnatural settings (clinics and labs) and with EF measures that are largely "cold" cognitive in nature that would miss this aspect of functioning or detect only the smallest instances of its degradation. Dimond (1980) makes a special point of noting the hundreds of cases of PFC injury that did not manifest many of the changes in cold cognition or mental functioning attributed to this region by others except for marked changes in planning and social functioning (pp. 505–508).

Eslinger (1996) in particular would later take up this call for the importance of EF (the PFC) in managing the social conduct of the individual. He argued that EF contains "social executors" that each serve certain social functions: (1) social self-regulation: processes needed to manage the initiation, rate, intensity, and duration of social interactions; (2) social self-awareness: knowledge and insight about oneself and the impact of one's behavior on others in social settings; (3) social sensitivity: the ability to understand another's perspective, point of view, or emotional state (similar to empathy); and (4) social salience: regulation of somatic and emotional states that impart a sense of meaningfulness to social situations and to specific individuals within that situation (p. 390).

In contrast to most modern cognitive views of EF, Eslinger (1996) viewed the social disability arising from EF impairment as frequently being the most distinctive feature beyond just the cold cognitive impairments. He states, "Yet there is no comprehensive model of executive function that addresses the interrelationship of cognitive and social aspects of behavior, including the various impairments that can occur" (p. 389). He lists the following as some of the social deficits arising from PFC (hence EF) damage: demanding and self-centered behavior, lack of social tact and restraint, impulsive speech and actions, disinhibition (of immediate self-interests), apathy and indifference, and lack of empathy, among others.

More recently, Rossano (2011) similarly bemoaned the dearth of references to the importance of social and emotional factors in studies and reviews on cognitive control, or EF, and its evolution. He reviewed anthropological evidence on the importance of both social and emotional functioning in the evolution of cognitive control in primates and especially humans. His review indicated that "theories of cognitive control are likely to be seriously incomplete unless they incorporate relevant social/emotional factors" (p. 238).

Absent these rare voices concerning the importance of EF (the PFC) for social behavior, and the role of social/emotional factors in its evolution, one would have thought that the major deficits suffered by those with PFC injuries were largely cognitive or information processing in form. Anyone who has spent any time with patients with PFC injuries or spoken with their family members would find such cognitive deficits to be trivial in comparison to the major social impairments arising from such injuries. From this clinical (and familial) perspective, the view of EF offered by cognitive psychology or those wedded to EF test batteries is not worth having. Their contents are devoid of social relevance and context. It is axiomatic that we do not live alone—humans are a group-living social species. When we engage in EF, we do so not just aware of our long-term self-interests but with an awareness of and in the context of other self-interested self-regulating agents with whom we interact. EF occurs not only across time toward future goals but usually *among social others!*

The Overlooked Importance of Emotion and Motivation in EF

A further problem with most theories and definitions of EF is the relative dearth of attention given to emotional and motivational aspects of self-regulation, as Rossano (2011) above also noted. While this issue is certainly discussed by Luria (1966) and others who described the consequences of frontal lobe injuries in humans and primates (Damasio, 1994, 1995; Dimond, 1980; Fuster, 1997; Stuss & Benson, 1986), it has been largely ignored in most other conceptualizations of EF in the past 30 years. This is particularly so in accounts of EF using cognitive psychology and information-processing models. Exceptions have been Fuster's theory of cross-temporal synthesis (1997), Damasio's (1994) somatic marker theory, Stuss and Benson's (1986) hierarchical model, and my own hybrid model of EF (Barkley, 1997a, 1997b). None are based on the computer metaphor of brain functioning that underlies information-processing models of EF. Perhaps this neglect arises because computers do not have emotions that need self-regulating and do not have to self-motivate.

The neglect of emotion may also stem from the inherently greater difficulty in measuring emotional and motivational states relative to the enormous number of tests available for assessing the more "cognitive" features of EF, such as working memory. Emotions are motivational states that undoubtedly play an important role in evaluating and determining one's means (actions) and ends (goals) and their social appropriateness (Damasio, 1994). They will also contribute the drive, willpower, or self-motivation that will be needed to achieve them (Barkley, 1997b; Fuster, 1997; Stuss & Benson, 1986). The supposedly "cool" EF brain networks, such as working memory, planning, problem solving, and foresight, may provide for the "what, where, and when" of goal-directed action, but it is the "hot" EF brain network (Castellanos et al., 2006; Nigg & Casey, 2005) that provides the "why" or basis for choosing to pursue that goal in the first place and the motivation that will be needed to get there.

The Limitations of the Computer Metaphor of Brain Functioning for EF

The foregoing discussion suggests yet a further problem with contemporary cognitive views of EF, and especially those predicated on information-processing models of brain functioning. Using the computer as a metaphor for brain functioning has undoubtedly been of value in efforts to advance the understanding of neural circuitry and its likely functions. But it has its limits for brains. Moreover, it is, after all, just a metaphor. Appreciating some of the major differences between computers and brains is important. First, computers are designed, whereas human brains evolved; hence the architecture and functioning of each are likely to be quite different. Engineers designing computers can determine the most efficient and effective designs for both hardware and software to achieve the intended purposes to which computers are used. Natural selection, acting on brains, has no such plans and foresight to use in its sculpting of the brain. Consequently, a computer may be a marvel of efficient design. But a brain is a veritable Rube Goldberg device of adaptations cobbled together from what had been available for other functions previously but that may be diverted to another function under a change in environmental pressure (a new adaptive problem). Evolution can only work on what was previously available and gradually tweak previous mechanisms or adaptations for use in the new function to which it is being put. As such, an adaptation is a patchwork of kludges or solutions arising out of whatever pieces (functions) were around at the time, so to speak. We must therefore be prepared for the fact that the human brain may be a mixture of older or vestigial adaptive functions that may be less useful or even disadvantageous in modern environments. Yet it may also contain a mixture of new ones that may even now still be in the process of evolving toward greater efficiency and effectiveness. Not all PFC functions are likely to be presently adaptive or useful, and others may be frankly maladaptive in modern, industrialized environments.

A second major distinction between computers and brains is that computers are passive whereas human brains are not. The computer metaphor portrays the brain as if it were software and hardware; given a certain input, this "computer" moves the information through various stages of processing to produce the output that we see virtually automatically, like an automaton, industrial robot, or artificial intelligence creation. *This is a very passive view of the organism,* devoid of what makes living things unique—they are *self-interested agents!* They have basic motives preinstalled that serve to sustain their own life (appetitive and defensive/protective motives) and to reproduce (that is, to transmit their genes) into the next generation (sexuality and competition for mates). This blindness to *self-interestedness and its motives* is a glaring deficiency in contemporary EF models. A computer is not a self-interested, self-motivating, self-regulating entity; a human brain is.

Another feature of animal life is locomotion—animals move and act under their own power and must frequently be attentive to refueling and maintaining their vehicles. Nature does not automatically provide for the life-sustaining needs of a human; that person must interact in such a way with that environment to produce its sustenance. Computers are not self-interested, do not self-assemble, do not compete with other computers for resources or mating rights, and do not concern themselves with the source of their own fuel or the integrity of their hardware. Such motivational considerations from biological evolution are absent in the modern concepts of EF. Only Dimond (1980, p. 504) seems to have taken note of them and given them some importance in understanding the losses that occur in PFC damage—our social intelligence that is necessary to insure our survival and reproductive self-interests. Humans have motivations that computers do not.

Some EF perspectives do acknowledge that drive, motivation, and will are prefrontal functions and are a component of or enslaved by EF (Stuss & Benson, 1986). But even these few fail to note that this is the fuel tank of all future-directed action and the EFs that contribute to that action. Humans act, and they do so with purpose (intentionality; a future-directed stance). Those actions are initiated and sustained by drive, motivation, and will and by the self-interested motives to survive, nourish themselves, and reproduce themselves into the next generation. Absent an appreciation for such motives in human action, computer metaphors of EF will prove strikingly sterile and self-limiting in helping us to understand EF or the functions of the PFC.

The Installation of a "Central Executive" or Homunculus in EF: The Ghost in the Machine

The next important problem with theories and their conceptualizations of EF, again noted by Dimond (1980) and later others (Hayes et al., 1996), is attributing "a central executive" to the PFC. This was the initial mistake made by Pribram (1973), and it has been repeated since that first appearance of the term "executive" as applied to the PFC's functions. Saying that the PFC is the brain's executive installs a *deus ex machina*, a marionette operator, or homunculus (Grafman, 1995) into the PFC that serves to explain nothing and will eventually require its own explanation. Saying that the PFC is the brain's central executive merely begs the issue of just who or what is this wizard behind the curtain that is pulling all these levers in managing the lower level nonexecutive brain systems so as to direct behavior across time toward future goals. Just who or what is even choosing these goals, and for whom are they being chosen? It is surely not some little CEO of a large corporation or a symphony conductor installed in the brain, as suggested in the analogies so often used as exemplars of EF in the trade literature. Yet most models of EF include some thinly veiled reference to some sort of "mini-me" that is doing our bidding, as Hayes et al. (1996) noted.

Since its inception by Pribram more than 40 years ago, the issue of who or what is the central executive has been kicked down the road incessantly. But it must eventually be addressed. One can temporarily sidestep this issue as is evident in decisions by working memory scientists (Baddeley, 1986; Baddeley & Hitch, 1994; Goldman-Rakic, 1995) to intentionally ignore the nature of the "central executive." Instead they focus their research on the subordinate working memory systems that serve to hold in mind the information and goals that the central executive has chosen. Or the central executive is simply inferred from the shared variance between nonverbal and verbal working memory tests without actually defining it and assessing it directly (Rapport et al., 2008). Understanding the nature of working memory is clearly a laudable and worthy research goal. However, it does not get us very far in understanding the entity to which the working memory systems are said to be slave units. Who or what is determining the contents of working memory and the goals they serve?

The Missing "Self" in EF

Strikingly absent from most views of EF other than that of Stuss and Benson (1986) is a role of *the self* in these models. In my view, the conscious self IS the central executive. Each of us develops a conscious sense of self, and it is this conscious self that is serving as the executive. It is through our self-awareness/self-consciousness that our values and wants are consciously known to us, our goals (values or what we wish to pursue) are chosen by us, and the strategies that we will employ in these pursuits are selected by us. Who chooses? *I* do. What is to be valued and pursued? What *I* choose to do. How is it to be pursued? The way *I* decide to do so. The "*I*" has been almost entirely jettisoned from cognitive theories of EF, replaced by some unknown, undefined central executive holed up in some penthouse office suite in the frontal lobes. This conscious capacity to consider who and what we are, what we will value, and how and when it will be pursued originates in our self-awareness. It is the seat of human free will as philosophy has noted (our freedom to choose among various goals over various time periods and the means to attain those goals). Stuss and Benson (1986) were absolutely correct, I believe, in making this mental capacity the apex of their pyramid of the EF system and its components.

Freedom here does not mean random or uncorrelated decision making between values (goals) and their means–ends. Freedom or free will is a conscious generation of and consideration of the variety of options available to that individual over the longer term as capable of being conceived by the individual. It also includes the selection of which goals to pursue, how to pursue them, and when to do so. This active agency of the self exists in philosophy but seems lost to or intentionally avoided by the field of neuropsychology. Perhaps this is because it is seen as unscientific or just difficult to measure. But it is neither. Instead, cognitive neuropsychology's view of humanity is frankly not worth having—an Orwellian automaton of an information processor without a sense of self.

Alternatively, constructs can be proposed in a scientific analysis of an issue on the basis of reason, experience, and logic that cannot yet be measured objectively at the moment. Objective measurement is not a precondition of scientific theorizing; rather, it is just the eventual possibility of testability of the proposal. We know that self-awareness is a brain function (Stuss & Benson, 1986), that it is largely a function of the PFC and related networks, and that it can be neuroimaged (Herwig, 2010). And we have ample evidence that this sense of ourselves as an active, thinking–choosing agent can be diminished by brain injuries, especially to the PFC. This self, however, is often spoken of in the third person, if at all, in cognitive models of EF. Even then it is not obviously a part of a living self-conscious entity as seen, for example, in statements such as the following on the nature of EF: "it monitors and controls all the steps necessary for a correct solution" (Borkowski & Burke, 1996, p. 242). *It?*

We should immediately recognize that the "it" here is actually the "I." Efforts to strip the self and self-awareness from EF are unnecessarily sterile of what every human accepts as axiomatic and as common sense: I am the agent consciously deciding what it is that I will do. Others hold that "I" accountable for its actions precisely for this reason. A software program in a computer is incapable of being held legally accountable for its choice of actions, but a human can and should be held so accountable. One chooses what he or she will do and ought to do using one's self-awareness and sense of the future—the longer-term consequences that are likely to ensue for one's self and for others given the various choices under consideration. It is time to return the self to the construct of EF.

Overlooking the Bidirectional Influence of EF and Culture

One can recognize that EF is of exceptional social importance and likely arose to meet social adaptive problems, such as social interaction and self-defense, reciprocity, cooperation, and hence survival (Barkley, 2001). But this does not in and of itself directly recognize an important place of culture in either contributing to EF or being influenced by it. Culture is shared information. It is the result of people individually and collectively pursuing their goals and discovering new and better means of doing so. These means and ends may be recorded, codified, or in other ways stored by means that endure sufficiently to be shared horizontally across people and vertically across time (generations). People both create and adopt culture. Yet it is equally true that the existing culture influences the people who are immersed within and who actively adopt it. That is, the information, products, services, and other innovations stored and transmitted from prior generations or even from others currently existing can and are used by people to provide better means by which they can pursue their goals and general self-interests. This reciprocal influence between EF and culture goes virtually unnoticed in prior views of EF. But its existence is virtually self-evident, requiring only the evidence of one's senses and very existence to affirm its validity. There are parts of the PFC that both use and create culture. Yet this exceptionally important aspect of human activity gets virtually no attention in modern models of EF.

For example, the computer on which these sentences are being composed is a product of past and current EF by other humans of which I am the benefactor. The computer, a cultural product, provides a far better means of attaining my goal (writing this book) than was the case for prior generations or even for me two decades ago. Even so, the product of this interplay between me and computer (this book) is intended to further influence the existing culture and others by its information. Save for the work of Vygotsky (1962, 1978, 1987) and a few others, the reciprocal influence of EF and culture has been utterly absent from conceptualizations of EF. Yet this interplay is in serious jeopardy of perversion, reduction, or complete loss when injuries of the PFC (and its EF system) are sustained. Some mental mechanism must exist for humans to create culture and to benefit from, adopt, or be influenced by it. That mechanism, in my opinion, is the EF system, explaining (if such explanation were needed) why only humans have culture.

Why EF?: The Importance of Evolution in the Origins and Purposes of EF

All of the above problems, as serious as they are, pale when compared to the even larger problem: Why do we have EF? I have argued elsewhere (Barkley, 2001) that virtually all of the efforts to understand the EF system and its components have ignored their likely evolutionary origins and purposes. The same has largely proven true in the literature on cognitive control (Rossano, 2011), an alternative term for EF in information-processing research. This is undoubtedly due in part to the legacy of adopting cognitive tests and their constructs in trying to study EF. It may also be the result of widespread ignorance of the theory of evolution among neuropsychologists and hence their neglect of its importance for understanding the nature of EF. But neuropsychology is a subspecialty of biology as much as of psychology, and the governing paradigm in biology is evolution. Yet one is hard pressed to find any mention of it in any treatise on EF by neuropsychologists, except vaguely by Dimond (1980) and more explicitly in a trade book by Gazzaniga (1998).

The theory of evolution provides a means by which one can understand the functional mechanisms that species have evolved to deal with problems they encounter in their environment—these functional mechanisms are their adaptations. The EF system is a complex functional mechanism that seems to have been designed for a purpose—it and the PFC that gives rise to it are costly. Such costly adaptations do not arise in evolution without providing their owners with some benefit to their survival, chances of reproduction, and inclusive fitness (the likelihood that their genes and those shared with relatives get into the next generation). EF is an adaptation that has evolved to solve a problem or set of problems faced by those few species that possess it. This is not a *non sequitur*—EF may have evolved to solve social problems. Humans are a social species, and living with other genetically related and unrelated individuals poses problems (and opportunities) for members of that species. There is a daily need to look ahead and anticipate what others are likely to do in the context of pursuing one's self-interests. We can rightly ask what specific adaptive problems the EFs evolved to solve in the environmental niche in which humans live. It surely was not sorting cards. Given that the vast majority of species do not possess this adaptation, it is highly unlikely to be necessary for surviving and reproducing on this planet. If it were, many species would have converged on it as an adaptive means of addressing problems in coping with the physical environment, such as has happened with the repeated evolution of eyes. It is highly likely that the EF system exists to assist humans with their social existence and its associated problems and opportunities. To what extent it is a result of either natural selection or sexual selection, or both (Miller, 1998), is of less concern here than that it is an adaptation that enhances either survival or reproduction, or both.

The answer as to why humans have EF may come from considering other species that have rudimentary prototypes of EF. Chimpanzees and dolphins seem to have a nonverbal working memory system, as do some species of monkeys, though far less developed. One thing that these species have in common is that they are social creatures. Unlike some group-living species of mammals and insects, chimpanzees, dolphins and some monkeys live in groups with individuals to whom they are not strongly genetically related. Where genetic relationships are high, cooperation with the group and mutual self-interest can arise by genetic (natural) selection, as members of the group are virtual clones of each other and thus have a highly shared genetic self-interest. But social primates often live in groups with others to whom they may be only modestly genetically related or not at all. The particular behaviors known to exist in the social primates (and dolphins) that deserve consideration as possible reasons for EF are reciprocal exchange (trading behavior, and especially delayed exchanges), social competition, social cooperation or mutualism (social symbiosis), and the protoethics and morality that exist to facilitate it. Both delayed reciprocal exchange (giving up a resource now to be repaid later) and cooperation (acting together to achieve goals not possible by an individual) require a sense of time, a means of evaluating the discount of delayed payments or other benefits, and a means of subordinating immediate self-interests to future benefits. Without a capacity to conceive of the longer term, these volitional forms of behavior are not possible. As already noted, it is precisely such behavior that is grossly impaired in individuals with damage to the PFC.

The species that have a proto-EF system also engage to a certain extent in imitation learning (a form of experiential or behavioral plagiarism). They possess a mirror neuronal system in the PFC that is highly specialized for this purpose. In humans, in particular, there is a dominant or prepotent response to overtly imitate another's actions, and it must be actively inhibited from being publicly expressed—the neuronal firing patterns that match the actions being watched are activated, but their release to the musculoskeletal system is inhibited. This instinct to imitate the actions of another can be partially disinhibited when working memory load increases because that increasing demand on the EF system undermines the executive inhibition of the habit of spontaneous imitation (van Leeuwen, van Baaren, Martin, Dijksterhuis, & Bekkering, 2009). The instinct to imitate is also likely to be disinhibited when the PFC is damaged (Luria, 1966).

The capacity to use the witnessing of another's experiences for one's own self-improvement is a tremendously useful adaptation among social species in which members compete against each other for resources. Humans also take imitation to an even higher level, which is vicariously learning to do the opposite of what one has seen another do. Vicarious learning is a particularly useful adaptation when it comes to learning from the mistakes made by others, some of which can be injurious or even lethal. It is self-evident that more learning occurs in response to errors than to successes. This must be immeasurably more so if one can profit from the mistakes made by others by observing their actions, the consequences, and then suppressing one's own predispositions to do the same. The inability to act in opposition to information and actions perceived in the sensory fields is a classic symptom of PFC damage (Luria, 1966; Stuss & Benson, 1986). The capacity to mentally represent information (working memory) allows an individual to wrest control of moment-to-moment behaving and even to act in opposition to what is seen.

There may be other social problems that the EF system has evolved to solve (Rossano, 2011). These may include theory of mind (anticipating that another also has a mind and especially an EF system and acting accordingly) and empathy (Grattan, Bloomer, Archambault, & Eslinger, 1994). These functions may even be facilitated by or even based on covert imitation. But the functions of delayed reciprocal exchange, social competition, social cooperation, and imitation and vicarious learning may have been the initial ones that kicked off the evolutionary expansion of the PFC in primates and especially humans. Only the first would be needed to veer human evolution down the path to the others, I believe (Barkley, 1997b, 2001). They are well worth our consideration in understanding EF. Performing a digit span backward task is trivial in comparison to these social functions and is surely not the adaptive problem the EF system evolved to solve.

Why does EF exist? What is it for? Isn't this why scientists have been studying the functions of the PFC for more than 160 years? After all, when you finally figure out what the PFC does, doesn't this invite the next question of why it does those things; why it exists? Understanding the possible adaptive problems in primate and human life that the PFC/EF system evolved to solve is the only way to answer these questions. This book will make an attempt to do so. It surely will not give definitive answers to these questions, but it can suggest some likely directions worthy of further research.

Conclusions and Specific Aims

This chapter has identified at least four serious interrelated problems in the field of EF in modern neuropsychology. This book aims to address these problems. The first difficulty is that the term "EF" lacks an operational definition that can serve to determine which human mental faculties should be graced with the moniker "executive" and which should not. The view that EF is maintaining goal-directed problem solving (Welsh & Pennington, 1988) or that it is those "skills necessary for purposeful, goal-directed activity" (Anderson, 1998, p. 319) will not suffice to meet this need—not when the neuropsychological processes needed to maintain problem solving toward a goal are incompletely or poorly specified or when the word "skills" can include 15 to 33 components. Moreover, use of the term *skill* is misleading as that is something one learns, like reading and writing, not an inherent neuropsychological capacity of the individual as EF is often represented as being in the literature. An operational definition of EF will be offered here that makes this task a relatively easier one. Meanwhile, I will accept as my starting point for defining EF the most commonly agreed upon feature of it as noted in the survey of neuropsychologists by Eslinger (1996)—EF is self-regulation. I will expand on this idea in subsequent chapters.

The second problem area is that current theories of EF have drifted away from capturing the characteristics of patients with PFC injuries or disorders of this "executive" brain, including their marked problems in emotional, social, economic, and moral domains, among others. Cognitive psychometrically based models of EF are common at this time. It is the aim of this book to propose a theory of EF that can unite these various levels of symptoms and deficits. Along the way, the third set of problems characterizing modern models of EF will also be addressed. The social purposes of EF will be placed at center stage in the higher levels of the theory proposed here. The important role of emotion regulation and self-motivation will also be explained and made an equally important component of EF, as are cold cognitive components such as planning and working memory. The computer metaphor of EF possessing a central executive or ghost in the machine will be abandoned here in favor of an acting self that ponders choices, makes decisions, and enacts those decisions over extensive periods of time and large social networks. The bidirectional nature of culture, unnoticed in modern cognitive models of EF, will be a major element in the extended EF phenotype to be discussed here.

The fourth problem of why humans have EF will be addressed by taking an evolutionary stance toward EF as an adaptation or suite of adaptations necessary for solving problems that arose in human social life. Concepts in evolution will be borrowed for any insight they may give into the reasons for the existence of EF. Three such major concepts are developed in the next chapter. The first is selfish gene theory, which explains why all living things are at their core self-interested replicators. To understand EF, we will have to take the individual's self-interests into account. What does EF do for the survival and reproductive and inclusive fitness of its owner? The second equally important concept is that of the extended phenotype as opposed to the conventional view of phenotypes. The latter represents simply a physical or behavioral trait of the organism. In contrast, Dawkins (1982) discusses how organisms in biological evolution possess phenotypes that produce effects at distances over space and time well beyond their skins. Phenotypic traits have effects that impact not just the immediate spatial and temporal environment but that also radiate outward from the organism. These effects may extend far beyond the proximal physical distance and short durations typically considered in the notion of a phenotype. In some cases, these effects may radiate outward for miles and over months or even years. Such effects are subject to natural selection and may even be the basis of the various adaptations of a species. No other species has altered the physical environment to such a degree, at such great spatial distances, and over such long spans of time as have humans. Humans not only adapt to their environments as do others species, but they adapt their environments to them—and they do it using EF. Such alterations to the environment can be studied for their value as part of the human EF phenotype. The concept of the extended phenotype will be considered in detail in the next chapter along with the third important concept, "universal Darwinism." The process of Darwinian evolution is now thought to be at work in the universe wherever information about the environment is found to have accumulated. Although genetics is the level at which it is best understood, it likely extends up to five levels beyond that one.

An extended phenotypic model of EF will also be able to address the second of our problems with EF—how to assess it. That model of EF will show why putative tests of EF are largely not related to EF as used in daily life activities and are not predictive of functioning in domains of major life activities that should be rife with EF. A hierarchical model of the extended phenotype of EF can explain how this glaring deficiency in EF tests can arise. Chapters 3 through 8 detail the hierarchical levels of the extended EF phenotype and discuss how the effects of those levels radiate outward and upward.

At this time neuropsychologists and other neuroscientists, such as those working on the role of EF in ADHD, are pursuing "endophenotypyes." These are presumably those psychological functions that seem closest to the brain's neural activity and so are closest to the genes and their proteins that serve as initial and intermediate pathways, respectively, to the EF behavioral phenotype. Although this goal is commendable in that it hopes to yield a better understanding of PFC disorders such as ADHD and of the EF deficits associated with them (Castellanos et al., 2006; Castellanos & Tannock, 2002), it is incredibly limited in scope.

I am asking you to look in the opposite direction. I am encouraging you to start with a given set of human mental functions comprising EF and look outward as to how they impact the individual's behavior, daily functioning, social relations, cooperative ventures, economic transactions, and even moral, legal, occupational, child-rearing, and community activities.

2

The Extended Phenotype

A Foundation for Modeling
Executive Functioning

Chapter 1 identified a number of problems in the definition, conceptualization, and measurement of EF, including the lack of an evolutionary stance toward its existence. I believe that these problems can be addressed by viewing EF as an extended phenotype (Dawkins, 1982)—a suite of neuropsychological abilities that create profound effects at a considerable distance and across lengthy time spans from the genotype that initially forms them.

The concept of an extended phenotype may not, in itself, be a testable idea (Dawkins, 1982). Instead, it is more a point of view, a new way of seeing what already is known about a species and how to understand and organize that knowledge. From such a change in perspective can come a richer understanding of the phenotype of a species and a firing up of the imagination that can lead to new ideas, theories, and even hypotheses to test that would not have been considered had not one's point of view changed.

The same is true for selfish gene theory (Dawkins, 1976), which shifts from the individual's or group's point of view to the gene's view of life. All a gene does is copy itself. Yet to see this activity as a form of selfishness, or better yet self-interestedness, provides a stunning change in perspective about genes and the organisms they build. From it numerous hypotheses have emerged concerning intergene competition, conflict, cooperation, and the conditions needed for such cooperative activities to evolve and stabilize. The emergent consequences of this change

37

in viewpoint for understanding genetic evolution and the behavior of organisms continue; yet the viewpoint itself is only a metaphor and so is not testable.

It is this type of change in perspective about EF that I seek to present, not only to address the problems with the concept of EF as described in Chapter 1 but also to fire the imaginations of those who study EF. By changing perspective, what is known will not just be seen differently, but new ideas about EF and new hypotheses can be formulated and tested that would not have previously been imagined.

In this chapter, I start by describing the conventional view of a phenotype and then continue with the extended phenotype as it is used in biological evolution. Selfish gene theory is very much a part of the extended phenotype. I then turn to the contemporary view that Darwinian evolution exists at multiple levels beyond genetics; it applies wherever information about the environment has accumulated.

The Conventional View of the Phenotype

From Genes to Proteins to Structures/Functions

It is common to view a phenotype as the physical structure of a plant or animal that arises from the translation of its genetic make-up (genotype) interacting with the immediately surrounding environment. The conventional view of a phenotype typically ends at the external shell or skin of the organism. When we speak of a human's phenotype, we typically describe hair, skin, and eye color, shape of the face, texture of the skin and hair, configuration of the teeth, the forward-facing placement of the eyes, height, body mass, upright posture and bipedal gait, structure of the appendages, opposable fingers and thumb, and so on. All are believed to be the outward expressions of differences among people and across species in their genes or suites of genes—their genotypes. This conventional view of a phenotype is exemplified as

genes → proteins and enzymes → structures and their functions

From Genes to Behaviors

Just as much a part of any phenotype, yet less likely to be included within the conventional view, are certain types of species-typical behavior. Many behavioral traits or predispositions have genetic contributions to them (Dawkins, 1982). Whenever a feature of an organism is affected to any degree by genetic variation (heritability), it can be shaped and molded by natural selection. This is no less true of behavior than of eye color. Many behavioral patterns are part of the human phenotype (Pinker, 2002). Changes in behavior frequently occur in an individual member of a species that may be beneficial to its survival and reproductive fitness. To the extent that this change is based on genetic mutation or variation, natural selection can further shape and mold the behavioral phenotype across subsequent generations. The end result is a genetic predisposition to behave in certain ways in environments that were routinely encountered by previous generations of the species. Should this behavioral change become sufficiently stable over time and across generations so as to benefit the reproductive and inclusive fitness of the individuals and their offspring that inherit it, the change may eventually sweep through the subsequent population of that species and become a common behavioral trait in its standard phenotype—a process known as Baldwinian evolution (named after the eminent psychologist James Mark Baldwin, who first proposed it; see Richards, 1987, and Wozniak, 2009). The study of such evolved behavioral patterns and their supporting mental modules are now the well-established field of evolutionary psychology (Barkow, Cosmides, & Tooby, 1992). Indeed, many species with nervous systems adjust their behavior as a function of the system's consequences, as in Skinnerian learning; this learning capacity is a product of evolution acting on the genes that build and operate such a nervous system. The enhanced survival value of behavioral sensitivity to consequences may explain the very existence of complex nervous systems that learn from the mistakes they produce. The notion that human behavioral patterns may have some genetic basis to them has led to an expansion of the conventional phenotypic view of late to include behavior, as represented below:

genes → proteins and enzymes → (neural) structures and functions → behavioral traits

But this is still a conventional view, even if modernized to include the last zone of behavioral traits.

An Extended Phenotype

From Genes to Environmental Artifacts (Inanimate Objects)

We accept the notion that genes can have effects on physical structural differences among people and between species. We have just seen that genes can also influence differences in the behavior of individuals to the degree that such differences are in any way affected by genetic differences, no matter how small. What may be harder to grasp is the idea that the inanimate artifacts created by the behavior of members of a species can also be just as readily attributed to its phenotype. For instance, a difference in a gene can affect the perception of certain colors, and therefore it influences the color of stones or twigs an organism such as an insect or bird may use to create its dwelling or nest. Any feature of that dwelling, such as color, or even the dwelling's very existence, may be considered an extension of its phenotype if those features in any way contribute to any change in survival or reproductive success. The organism's gene for color perception is also, by extension, a gene that can influence the behavior of color selection of materials in the environment, and so it can be viewed as a gene for dwelling color (or structure) in that organism. When the coloring of the dwelling has an impact on the survival and reproduction of that organism, that makes it a functional feature of the extended phenotype of that gene and the individual (body) in which that gene is housed (Dawkins, 1982). It is not at all farfetched to consider examples where the success of birds or animals in attracting mates is in large part a consequence of the physical displays and artifacts they have created through their behavior, as in the bower of the bower bird or the nest of a squirrel or the dam of a beaver. Such environmental rearrangements of the material world and the artifacts so created can therefore be viewed as extensions of an organism's genotype and thus be part of its phenotype. It is here, then, that we part company with the conventional view of a phenotype and enter the view of the extended phenotype (Dawkins, 1982). That view can be represented as

genes → proteins and enzymes → structures and functions → behavioral traits → artifacts

The genes involved have created an effect at a spatial distance much further removed from the genotype or even from the structural anatomy of the eye. The effects have moved outward to include the artifacts created by the behavior that a structure, such as the eye and its related brain region, has influenced. In fact, the selection pressure in evolution that may have driven the evolution of color perception, eye structure, and its genes may well have been at the level of these artifacts and their consequences for mating and survival. As Dawkins explained it, there is no difference between a gene that results in a blue pigment in a bird's feathers that enhances its sexual attractiveness to mates and one that results in a bird painting its bower with a blue pigment that achieves the same effect on its likelihood of mating. The fact that the former is a conventional view of a phenotype and the latter an extended phenotypic perspective is a distinction without a difference. Yet, few if any would have realized this had Dawkins not switched points of view to consider the long reach of the gene—that genetic effects can occur at distances that lie outside of organisms, including the artifacts they create.

It is likewise just as easy to see that genetic differences between spiders, even in the same species, may influence the manner in which they build their webs. Idiosyncrasies in web structure may be to the advantage or detriment of the spider's surviving and reproducing, and even influence the survival of her offspring in the egg sack housed nearby that web. The web, though outside the body, is just as much a feature of the spider's phenotype as its behavior, body structure, and genotype that led through this pathway to the external artifacts. It's a phenotype all the way out. The same can be said of humans. To the degree that any of the artifacts we create, such as shelters, tools, and clothing, are a conse-quence of genetic variation, those artifacts are just as much a part of the human phenotype as are the behavioral traits that led to their creation and the brain structures and functions that produce those behavioral traits. In fact, such artifacts may have influenced the evolution of those structures and their functions (Taylor, 2010).

From Genes to Shared Inanimate Artifacts, Cooperatively Created

Now let's extend this perspective even further out from the genotype. Consider instances in which colonies of organisms such as social insects act together to create a mound, beehive, underground series of tunnels, or other structure. The fact that these structures were not created by a single individual but by a cooperative group activity does not change the fact that the structure is part of that social organism's phenotype. Genes exist for such cooperative behavior among highly genetically similar, if not identical, social species (Dawkins, 1982). In species such as ants, termites, or prairie dogs, variations in those genes that contribute to cooperative mound or nest building may lead to variations in mound or nest structure. These structures can be considered just as much a part of the phenotype as the bodily shape or social behavior of that organism. A behavioral geneticist would have no difficulty in any of these instances of examining genetic variation in that species as it may be related to variation in such environmental artifacts. That is to say, there is genetic variation in the species for the structure of its nests or mounds. He or she would be correct to conclude that the artifact is an extended phenotypic effect of such genetic differences, even though the artifacts exist some distance from the individual organism's genes or body and arose from a cooperative venture (Dawkins, 1982). This, as Dawkins reasoned, could lead to an entirely new subspecialty of behavioral genetics—that of artifact genetics.

The difference from the preceding level is simply that the artifact (mound) was created by a cooperating group of individuals that have a strongly shared genetic self-interest rather than by a single organism. This act of cooperation among individuals is no less a function of genetic influence than was the teaming up of genes to create chromosomes in early evolution, the teaming up of two different prokaryotic cell types to form more complex eukaryotic cells, the teaming up of such cells to form multicellular bodies, and on to the teaming up of multiple individual bodies to form a community. All forms of cooperation at any of these evolutionary transitions arise from a shared self-interest in which greater survival advantages can be had at the higher level of cooperation than at the lower level of individual units (Maynard Smith & Szathmary, 1999; Michod, 1999). All can be considered phenotypic effects of genes and suites of genes that form genotypes and hence phenotypes. In this instance, social behavior yields shared artifacts, and both can be considered a phenotypic effect of genotypic differences. The extension might look something like the following, with the same string of effects occurring in multiple individuals working together to create a product, such as in a social species:

genes → proteins and enzymes → structures and functions →
behavioral traits → shared artifacts

We have now broached the possibility that some forms of social behavior and the artifacts such cooperative acts produce can be part of the extended phenotype of that social species. There is no reason this might not be as true of humans as it is of other social organisms. It even opens up the potential that humans acting cooperatively to create shared artifacts make those artifacts part of the surrounding culture. This would make culture part of the human extended phenotype—an important point to be discussed in detail in later chapters. However, it is easier to understand the origin of shared genetic self-interests in the case of social insects, as noted above. Such insects are highly genetically related, if not outright clones of each other. That makes it much easier for genes affecting altruistic and cooperative behavior to arise and spread by natural selection among members of the species.

The origin of shared self-interests among cooperating organisms that have *little* or *no* shared genetic self-interest (they are not relatives or only distantly so) requires some other explanation for its basis. The answer, I believe, lies in the nature of EF. It will be discussed briefly below and in more detail in later chapters. Suffice to say here that the general conditions necessary for cooperation to arise at any transition in evolution, including that of human groups, are quite similar. We will look for those conditions at that level at which the human EF phenotype engages in cooperative ventures with other humans. Its motive, as always in cooperative activity, is self-interest. But when individual self-interests at any level of biology converge sufficiently to be shared across individuals living in close proximity to each other, the potential or opportunity for cooperative (mutually beneficial) activity among those individuals arises (Michod, 1999).

From Genes to Effects on Other Animate Entities (Organisms)

Let us consider another variation on the theme of extended phenotypic effects on the environment. In the above case, the extended effect was on the creation of inanimate artifacts, either solo or shared. There is absolutely no reason why such extended phenotypic effects could not occur on animate objects, which is to say other living organisms. In point of fact, there are many reasons why such extended effects would and could be included in the extended phenotype of that organism. The environment of a species is not just made up of the inanimate material world; it often comprises other living things. To the extent that genetic variation can result in behavioral traits and artifacts that can be used to influence the structure, functions, and behavioral traits of another organism, such effects can also be incorporated into the concept of an extended phenotype.

Take as an example tape worms or fluke worms. These worms may, through their behavior and life cycle, come to invade the bodies of intermediate and final hosts. After invasion, they reproduce using the resources of their host and migrate to parts of the organism that can eventually cause the hosts to excrete them. As their hosts move about, these parasites travel with them. The host thereby deposits these parasites much farther across spatial distances than the worms could have achieved on their own. By doing so, the worms more easily spread to other intermediate and final hosts. And should the host be a social species, its social interactions with proximate members serves to create an even greater opportunity for the worms to spread to new hosts. The extended phenotype of the worm has now literally jumped the gap between it and another organism. In this case, it did so by invasion of the other organism. This gap between organisms and how it gets crossed is often ignored in the conventional view of a phenotype. The phenotype of the worm has invaded the phenotype of another organism and used that organism for its own welfare. This extended phenotype can now look like this:

genes → proteins and enzymes → structures and functions →
behavioral traits → other organisms

What we have witnessed in this case or in other parasitic relationships is the overlap of radiating effects of one extended phenotype on that of another—in this case through the physical invasion of one phenotype by another. In so doing, genes in one organism produce favorable effects for it by manipulating the structures and functions of other organisms—in this case by being inside of them. By this means, the parasite enhances its survival and reproduction at the expense of the other organism. The invasion and manipulation of the host organism by the parasite are extended phenotypic effects of that parasite's genotype. The changes produced in the structures or internal functions of the host organism by the invader are just as much a part of the invader's phenotype as is its own bodily structures and their functions.

From Genes to the Behavior of Other Organisms

It is now but another small step in the outward radiation of an extended phenotype to show how genes or genotypes of one organism can manipulate not just the structures and internal functions of a host organism through such invasion, but also its *behavior* to the advantage of the parasite. Such behavioral changes can also be to the parasite's own benefit. The rabies virus is Dawkins's (1982) example of this process. This virus infects its warm-blooded host, reproduces using host resources, and migrates to other organ systems, such as the salivary glands, and especially to the host's brain. The virus then alters the host's brain in such a way as to initially increase affectionate behavior, as in an infected dog increasing its licking of other dogs or its caretaker thereby spreading the virus contained in the salivary glands to other creatures. The brain alterations eventually result in increased wandering behavior and aggression against other animals, usually through biting them. The virus has now caused the host to attack and bite other creatures and, through the bite, to transmit the virus to another host. This is an instance among many in which organisms behave in ways that manipulate the structure, function, *and behavior* of other organisms to their own advantage or self-interests (Dawkins, 1982). Now the extended phenotypic chain looks like this:

genes → proteins and enzymes → structures and functions →
behavioral traits → other organisms → other organisms' behavior

Jumping the Gap between Organisms without Host Invasion

In the above example, one organism affects other organisms and their behavior through invasion of a host. But there are other ways to manipulate one organism to the advantage of another short of all-out invasion of the host. For instance, pheromones or other chemical signals can be released or even projected by an organism so as to come into contact with the host. Such chemicals can then enter the recipient through its skin or sense receptors and so manipulate the recipient to the signaler's advantage. Such manipulation can be by direct chemical reactions or simply through altering the perceptual signals of sense receptors. An example given by Dawkins (1982) is of a species of mice in which some males emit a pheromone that causes pregnant females to abort that pregnancy. This brings the female into estrus quickly and so gives the male the opportunity to eliminate the offspring of a male rival and impregnate the female with his own sperm. The gap between the two organisms was crossed without direct invasion of one by the other. The end result is the same as if invasion had occurred—the manipulation of a recipient by a signaling organism to the signaler's advantage.

The signals, however, do not have to be chemical in nature. They could be structural alterations in the appearance of the originating organism that, when perceived by the recipient, makes the recipient more or less likely to behave in ways favorable to the signaler. This can be seen in cases of brilliant colorations of an organism that alter the behavior of another, as in courtship displays, or via camouflage colorations that change the likelihood of the organism being detected by its predators. A common example is the brilliant coloration of a peacock's tail that reliably signals the health of the individual (that they can carry the burden of a handicap without reducing their health) and thereby makes the female peahen more likely to breed with the signaler (Zahavi

& Zahavi, 1997). Such signals are an extra phenotypic burden but may still evolve because they influence mating opportunities with peahens by signaling that the male is healthy. Indeed, much variation in physical phenotypic traits may arise from such sexual signaling, known as sexual selection—a special case of natural selection. A large number of human traits may well have evolved to alter the behavior of the opposite sex, usually to increase mating opportunity (Zahavi & Zahavi, 1997).

The gap between signaler and recipient can also be crossed using sound (such as vocalizations) produced by the signaling organism. The signals alter sense receptors (in this case, those for hearing) to produce a change in the recipient that is favorable to the self-interests of the sender. A vocalization is no different in the end than a chemical pheromone sprayed across the gap between organisms or a chemical hormone released inside a host after it has been invaded. Vocalization can profitably be viewed analogously to that of a drug that has affected the body or brain of the recipient. It is useful to examine the various forms of communication between organisms, including human language, for this possibility; they may have arisen at least in part as a means of manipulating the function and behavior of other organisms to the transmitter's own self-interests. Those manipulations could be for the good of both parties and their kin (mutually symbiotic) or work just as well to manipulate an unrelated individual to the sender's own advantage (parasitic). All means of gap-crossing achieve a similar end: to manipulate the structure and function and even behavior of the recipient organism for the self-interests of the signaler. Our sequential diagram of the extended phenotype might now resemble this:

genes → proteins and enzymes → structures and functions →
behavioral traits → signaling devices →
other organisms' structures and functions → other organisms' behavior

All this leads to the fascinating possibility that there is genetic variation in the initiating organism that is related to structural and behavioral variation in the host or recipient organism. This can occur not only when the parasite invades the body of the host organism but even when the gap to the other organism is crossed by various signaling methods. Differing versions of genes in the initiator organism give rise to variations in its effectiveness at manipulating the structure, functioning, and behavior of the host or recipient organism, and those variations are subject to inheritance and natural selection in that initiator. To put it simply, there are genes in one organism for the behavior of another organism in which those genes are not housed and for whose benefit they are not working. This leads to Dawkins's (1982) fascinating central theorem: "An animal's behavior tends to maximize the survival of the genes 'for' that behavior, whether or not those genes happen to be in the body of the particular animal performing it" (p. 233).

A behavioral geneticist studying the phenotype of the initiating organism would assign this variation in the behavior of the recipient as obviously one of genetic contribution rather than that of common or unique environment in that initiator. But that same geneticist focusing on the variation in the behavior of the host or recipient organism would have to classify some of that variation as arising from "the environment" because it is not a consequence of the genes housed in the host organism. Yet that environmental component is, in the end, a genetic contribution; the fact that it arises from genetic variation in another organism makes it no less genetic in nature. It has only arisen in a separate genotype. Thus, when behavioral geneticists go about studying human psychological phenotypic traits, such as EF or its disorders, they should pay some heed to this possibility. That is, they should consider the possibility that some of the trait variation they have parsed into an environmental component for one organism could be arising from genetic variation in other humans that are manipulating that host for their own benefit or have tried to do so in the past history of the species.

Reciprocal Influences between Extended Phenotypes

At the next step in the logical progression of this viewpoint, things can get even more interesting. Organisms that are being influenced by an initiator organism are not passive over evolutionary time. We can expect the recipient species to eventually evolve defenses against easy manipulation. This process can then lead to new counteroffensives eventually evolving in the initiator, and so on, like an arms race. Our immune system is just such a defense mechanism against the invasion of our bodies by parasites. Genotypes and their phenotypes of the host will be shaped and molded to protect the host's welfare, survival, and reproduction. Should such reciprocal effects between two types of organisms continue across generations, natural selection would result in the recipient organism having a reasonably successful, genetically mediated defense against manipulation by the initiator organism. Selection pressures on the initiator might then produce new ways to manipulate the other.

In short, an arms race ensues between host/recipient and parasite/manipulator, with each evolving new genetically mediated mechanisms for adapting to the latest response of the other. This leads to the fascinating likelihood that genes residing in one organism have modifying and mediating genes in a different organism that are in response to the phenotypic effects of the former organism. Similar extended phenotypic effects can be seen in the evolution of predator–prey relationships. Such arms races can result in a stalemate; an evolutionarily stable arrangement. This may last until a new change in either phenotype threatens this balance and ignites yet another round of evolution–counterevolution.

These phenotypic effects may be parasitic, as in the case of rabies or even that of the common cold that causes you to sneeze and so project it to another host that it may now infect. The counterreaction of the host comes through its immune system, at least initially. Defensive changes in other bodily functions and even in behavior may also ensue. Or the arrangement may be symbiotic, in which case both species appear to mutually benefit from the extended phenotypic effects each has on the other in their relationship. In all of these cases, the extended phenotypic effect would become bidirectional. Although it is possible for one organism to win this arms race and even eliminate the other organism, this is unlikely given that the initiating organism needs the one it is manipulating to survive and reproduce. If it is too successful at such manipulation to the point where the host or manipulated organism cannot survive or reproduce, then it has eliminated its meal-ticket, so to speak, and will be adversely affected in its own survival and reproduction. More common is the situation of a stalemate or stable strategy that coexists between the two species.

Notice that the effect of each organism on the other could occur at any link in the chain of phenotypic effects. It should be remembered that the reciprocal influence of organisms on each other, including the arms races, stalemates, or symbiotic balances, are actually between the genes that created these organisms and not the gene vehicles, their bodies (Dawkins, 1976, 1982).

This extended phenotypic effect of one organism on another and the latter's reciprocal effects in return are not limited to bacteria or viruses or social insects. There is no conceivable reason why this cannot be the case in animals, mammals, primates, or even in human social interactions, relations, and networks, as it is in the rest of the living world. Bear this in mind as we later encounter the social zones of the extended phenotype of EF. Phenotypes may be shaped in part by the efforts of other individuals to manipulate us to their own benefit and our own social self-defense mechanisms that arise in response. Given the logical sequence of the argument laid out here for an extended phenotype, it is not a great stretch of the imagination to consider that human social conduct and communication, such as language, serve to manipulate the behavior of others to the advantage of our own self-interests (parasitic) or for mutual (symbiotic) self-interests (Barkley, 2001). Such social conduct and communication might be viewed usefully as the extended phenotypic effects of human EF phenotypes on each other.

The Living World: Overlapping Extended Phenotypes

It is not easy to know the extended phenotypic zone at which natural selection operates to produce a change in the underlying genotype. Natural selection may well be operating on effects of the phenotype that occur at some distances from that genotype and its vehicle, the body. Phenotypes can be considered to extend outward from organisms, like a series of concentric rings representing the widening fields of their radiating impact on features of the environment that may be distant in space and time (Dawkins, 1982). Some features of the environment are other living organisms and even other members of the same species. The living world resembles a web, a network of interconnected or interacting phenotypic effects, whether we consider it across all living things or just individuals within a particular species. The genes and genotypes of each organism radiate phenotypic effects that can overlap with similarly radiating effects from other organisms' genotypes and in which reciprocal influences occur among them.

While highly useful as a viewpoint in biology and the evolution of a species' phenotype, the extended phenotype (genetic effects-at-a-distance) is rarely considered in discussions of phenotypic traits in human psychology. Yet the concept may be very important in considering the evolutionary history of and basis for the emergence of any adaptive trait whether in biology or psychology. One of those traits may well include EF, as I argue in this book.

To end this brief summation of one of the most important modern concepts in biological evolution, I will let Dawkins speak for himself:

> I have a dim vision of phenotypic characters in an evolutionary space being tugged in different directions by replicators [genes] under selection. It is of the essence of my approach that the replicators tugging on any given phenotypic feature will include some from outside the body as well as those inside it. Some will obviously be tugging harder than others, so the arrows of force will have varying magnitude as well as direction. Presumably the theory of arms races . . . will have a prominent role to play in the assignment of these magnitudes. Sheer physical proximity will probably play a

role: genes seem likely, other things being equal, to exert more power over
nearby phenotypic characters than over distant ones. . . . But these will be
quantitative effects, to be weighed in the balance with other considerations
from arms race theory. Sometimes . . . genes in other bodies may exert
more power than the body's own genes, over particular aspects of the phenotype. My hunch is that almost all phenotypic characters will turn out
to bear the marks of compromise between internal and external replicator
forces. (1982, p. 248)

How Long Is the Reach of the Genes?:
The Boundary of the Extended Phenotype

How far out can phenotypic effects be extended without being absurd?
As illustrated by Dawkins (1982), does the footprint of a bird left behind
in the mud qualify as an extended phenotype of the bird? Or does the
fact that this footprint may affect single-celled organisms that populate
and reproduce in the small pool of water so created also qualify as
extended phenotypic effects of the bird? No, or at least probably not.
The phenotype can be said to extend only out to where it has some
effect on survival or reproduction of that genotype (its inclusive fitness).
That is where natural selection works—via differential rates of survival
and reproduction of genes and genotypes as a consequence of differences in genes and their extended effects. If it cannot be shown that the
footprint has such an effect on the bird's genotype, natural selection is
blind to it. Therefore, effects like the footprint in the mud left by the
bird are merely a by-product of the organism's phenotype, not a part of
it. The effect is of no use in our analysis as part of the bird's extended
phenotype because it has no consequences for the bird's survival and
reproduction.

In fact, this is one of the positive features of an extended phenotypic
analysis compared to a conventional one—the consideration of what
effects of an organism and its behavior on the environment including
other organisms might or might not qualify for phenotypic status. That
question is answered by studying what effects genes may have at a distance that impact their survival and reproduction and hence are subject
to the forces of natural selection to shape their evolution. It forces us to
look in places and at distances from organisms we might otherwise have
not thought to consider. One such place to look is human EF and its
extended effects into human daily functioning.

Where in the chain of phenotypic effects that a scientist may elect
to focus research is actually arbitrary. It is driven more by the particular

hypothesis being pursued with regard to that chain of effects. No level is necessarily more important or more likely to represent the phenotype (or be a gold standard) than any other. The decision of one scientist to focus on genetic variation in the phenotype of eyes at the level of the structural variation of the eye is no more or less likely to be the best approach than is the approach by one who studies variation in color perception that results from such structural variation. And that focus is no better than that of one who studies choices in apparel that may arise from such variations in perception. All are extended effects of the phenotype, and one level is no more phenotypic or genotypic than the others. Therefore, the argument by neuroscientists and neuropsychologists noted earlier that the best level on which to focus research on EF (or disorders like ADHD) is that of an endophenotype is baseless because it is arbitrary.

Studying this endophenotypic level of the phenotype may be interesting in its own right, provided that certain hypotheses under investigation warrant looking here. But this level of the extended phenotype is not the only level worthy of study. In fact, it may be that the very evolutionary basis for the existence of the phenotypic trait under investigation can actually be explained better by focusing on the effects it produces at a longer distance or in an outer zone of the radiating effects of the extended phenotype. For instance, studying the structures in male mice that create the abortion-inducing pheromone noted earlier may answer interesting scientific questions about glands and their bodily functions, but it does not explain why the pheromone evolved—it exists to abort fetuses in pregnant female mice. Only the extended phenotypic viewpoint, and not an endophenotypic one, would have provided that answer.

An Example of an Extended Phenotype

A useful example of an extended phenotype given by Dawkins (1982) is the impact of a beaver on the larger ecology of the region in which it lives. Many people may consider the phenotype of the beaver to be its mammalian physical features, especially its large front teeth, paddle-like tail, and other physical and behavioral traits that permit it to lead a partially aquatic lifestyle and to fell timber for use in making its lodge. But the beaver's physical and behavioral traits also have effects-at-a-distance (Dawkins, 1982). These traits must also be examined in understanding the entire phenotype and its evolutionary history. By dragging timber to a waterway, beavers create paths that make subsequent such efforts easier and so involve less energy expenditure (a good thing in evolutionary terms). These trails also produce effects on adjacent flora and fauna. Some of those changes may be of no consequence to beaver survival and reproduction, but some might. By building dams and homes on streams, beavers create ever widening ponds of still water. As Dawkins noted (1982), the size of the lake created by a beaver dam can be considered part of the extended phenotype of beavers because it does have an impact on beaver survival and reproduction. It likely arose through genetic variation in beaver behavior. Furthermore, these bodies of water not only make felled timber easier to transport by floating it to the nest/dam site, they also alter the adjacent flora and fauna of the region. Such alterations thereby produce effects on the locale from which the beaver and its offspring may prosper. There are also effects on other species that occupy that region and on the proximal ecological climate, such as in cloud formations, rainfall, and temperature among other effects on the physical environment. To the extent that any such changes in the environment feed back to benefit the beaver and its kin, they can be considered part of the extended phenotype of the beaver. The fact that the building of the dam and home was a cooperative effort of several beavers simply serves to bring socially cooperative behavior and its artifacts within the purview of an extended phenotype of a beaver. Thus, in studying the manner in which natural selection may be acting on a trait, researchers need to consider all phenotypic effects often at distances far removed from the gene and its bodily container. Researchers should not be so myopic as to focus only on those immediately visible physical attributes of the organism or the most spatially proximal and temporally immediate effects of its behavioral adaptations on the environment.

The Role of Universal Darwinism in the Human Extended Phenotype

One further set of evolutionary concepts is important for understanding the extended phenotype. Darwinian evolution is now thought to exist universally and is not limited to the genetic level, though that is the level at which it is best understood at this time. Evolution is seen as a general explanation for how information about the environment can accumulate (Campbell, 1960). *Anywhere in the universe that information about the environment (knowledge) can be found to have accumulated, it will have done so by a Darwinian process of evolution (replication with retention and environmental selection).*

The general algorithm (procedural steps) for how this happens is shown in Sidebar 2.1. Several different levels of evolution are now believed to exist, and each is partially dependent on and derived from the levels below it. These levels are genetic (slowest) (Dawkins, 1996; Ridley, Mark, 1996), operant conditioning (Skinner, 1981, 1984), vicarious or observational learning (Donald, 1991, 1993), mimetic–ideational (overt and covert rehearsal to the self, or simulation; Donald, 1991, 1993; Lumsden & Wilson, 1982), gestural communication/language (Blackmore, 1999; Dawkins, 1976), mental symbolic (simulation via internal language) (fastest) (Barkley, 1997b, 2001; Popper & Eccles, 1977), and cultural–artifactual (Durham, 1991). Each level relies on a different storage device to accumulate information, a different means of encoding that information, and a different mechanism to replicate it. Nevertheless, each is a specific instance of universal evolution. All of the steps in the algorithm exist at each of these levels.

Humans benefit from all levels and modes of inheritance (evolution) that result in the accumulation of information about the environment. Each level provides a progressively more rapid adjustment of the species or its individual members to changes in its environment. That is because at each new level, the time between trials is shortened considerably, permitting the testing of information against the environment to progress more rapidly. More trials can be executed in the same unit of time as we move up to each new level. The number of levels and modes of transmission are debatable and unimportant here. What *is* important is the existence of levels other than the genetic.

The general algorithm of evolution is important to understanding the extended phenotype of EF for two reasons. First, a large part of the EF phenotype is a result of evolution occurring at the level of genetics. Variation in EF is predicted here to be highly heritable, meaning that a substantial degree of individual differences in the psychological *capacities* involved in EF and its components are the result of differences in the genes. Second, multiple modes of inheritance based on the same general algorithm have arisen at least six more times beyond the genetic level. Several of these are intrapersonal in form and so contribute to or are components of EF (i.e., ideational and symbolic levels). Note that the levels alternate between the interpersonal and the intrapersonal. This may signal that the next level to evolve (if it has not already done so) is likely to be intrapersonal.

A distinctive feature of this view of the human extended phenotype is that it is dynamic, not static. At higher levels of universal informational evolution, the capacity for adapting to environmental change speeds up. The following looks more closely at the six levels beyond the genetic.

SIDEBAR 2.1. The Steps in the Evolution Algorithm

For any system of information to evolve, as in genetic evolution, it must involve at least eight processes:

1. *A storage device.* There must be a reliable storage device or memory base, that is, some means by which information can be reliably stored and accessed.

2. *A means of information encoding.* There must be a reliable means by which information can be coded into the storage device. In the case of biological evolution, this is just four little bits of information called nucleic acids which here we can simply call A, G, C, T.

3. *A means of replication (copying, trials).* At its core, the very essence of life is self-replication—making a copy of the initial information. For evolution to occur, there must be some means by which the information is copied (replicated). In the case of biology, the very first living molecule was the first one to copy itself. Each replication can be considered a trial in that the copy will be judged by the environment (see below) for its fitness or conformity to that environment—that is, its ability to continue its existence and replicate in it. Replication was the beginning of all knowledge acquisition and retention systems.

4. *Good but imperfect fidelity (of copying).* Replication must create a highly similar copy from its original. However, no copy will be perfectly identical to its original or template. Errors always creep into the copying process because the world changes from one moment to the next and those changes can affect the copying. But all that is needed is that the copy be good enough to work to serve its purpose—to replicate the information.

5. *Mistakes (mutations) must be made.* While this restates the above point that mistakes occur in the copying process, the emphasis here is that there can be no evolution if the copying is perfect every time. Fallibility (errors) is an essential ingredient in the evolution process. Such change in the information base is crucial; it created a new piece or arrangement of information that did not previously exist. It happens by accident and not by design, but it happens. Errors are ubiquitous in all of life. It is this blind, stupid, unconscious mistake-making that is the source of all new information, including that arising from human thinking. This point cannot be overemphasized. *Making mistakes is therefore absolutely crucial in the process of how evolution achieves new, more complex, and better adapted (efficient and functional) designs (the manifestations of the accumulated knowledge).* Most copying mistakes have no significant functional effect on the copy, and many mistakes may actually be detrimental. Indeed, some of them are absolutely destructive and may make the copy so deformed that it cannot do what it used to do. Its likelihood of survival (being repeated) is decreased, and it may not even last until the next copying takes place (it dies). But every once in a great while the mistake is an improvement to the original information base (design); it is useful for the design and its function.

It conforms better to reality. It need only be 1% of all mistakes—that's enough. And it will eventually result in improvements in the previous design because this new, more useful information (mutations) is replicated with the larger database that houses it and accumulates over time.

6. *A specific environment exists.* For information to exist, it must exist *somewhere.* That "where" is material reality. It is often called the environment, which just means a local region of reality. Every specific environment has specific characteristics that make it different from every other specific situation or setting.

7. *A selecting feature (an effect) of that environment.* Some aspect of the environment has to effect the likelihood that copies will survive or be destroyed in that environment. In this way, one or more specific characteristics of the environment serve as a mechanism for selection. This is why biological evolution is called natural selection. If the environment has absolutely no feature that has any influence on the survival of the copies, then no evolution will take place other than the piling up of mistakes over time in subsequent copies. If this goes on long enough, copying may no longer be possible. The information base is then in a sense dead; it is merely junk. But this is unlikely because specific settings often do have specific features that are going to have some effect on which copies have a better chance of being replicated the next time around. Combined with imperfect copying discussed above, the environment by its very nature selects the information (knowledge) that best conforms to it, and so over repeated trials it becomes closer and closer to conforming to reality (accuracy or truth value) with each trial. It is an automatic process. To the extent that environmental features have any effect on the copying process, they are acting (blindly) to select some strings or forms of information over others in the information base when the copying is taking place. Inherent in all material reality is this capacity to have a shaping or selective influence on any information that is being stored, copied, and thus tested within that environment. This selecting function of the environment can be thought of as **criticism.** It is the feedback from the environment concerning whether the information being tested better conforms or not to that environment, to reality. The more it conforms, the more *correct* it is and the less the environment *disagrees* with it. The less it conforms, the more the environment disagrees with it. This is a comparative process indicating how well the information or knowledge matches the environment. In a sense, it is about how well the information is modeling reality. In any particular trial, such criticism has the effect of making information less likely to survive to the next trial. Criticism is disagreement. Here then is another secret to the development of all knowledge anywhere in the universe: it must be *criticized!*

8. *Environmental change.* When something happens (it could be nearly anything), that changes the selecting feature of the particular environment (Step 7 above). That is all that is needed for one type of thing such as a species (information database) to become two different yet related things. In biology, this is the origin of new species emerging over repeated trials

(continued)

SIDEBAR 2.1. (*continued*)

from older ones. In animal learning, it is the origin of remarkably new and different behavior out of old behavior. In social learning, it is the creation of entirely new response patterns from those of others. And in cultural progress, it is the emergence of new cultural products from previous ones. In the case of conscious reasoning, it is developing remarkably new ideas, ways of doing things, action plans, and human products out of older related ideas.

• *Operant conditioning*. The evolution of Skinnerian (operant) learning in animals, for instance, created a second level of evolution that occurs within individuals and allows a more rapid adaptation to the environment and its changes than could occur at the genetic level alone. The phenotype of those species that learn by this method is more dynamic in that it permits more rapid adaptation of the organism under changing environmental conditions. It provides them with an additional degree of freedom, so to speak, from the tyranny of their genes; at this and each additional level of evolution, freedom evolves (Dennett, 2003). Yet this operant learning level is still partially dependent on the genes that produce nervous systems.

• *Vicarious learning*. I have previously argued that the evolution of vicarious learning provided the next level of evolution beyond the genetic and operant ones. Because of it, individuals no longer learned just by trial and error but could more rapidly adapt their behavior to the environment through observational learning (Barkley, 1997b). Vicarious learners are far more adaptive and hence dynamic. They can adapt more quickly because they benefit from everyone else's trial-and-error learning, not just their own. Vicarious learning provides another mechanism for the accumulation and replication of information. It thus represents yet another level of evolution. Moreover, it forms protoculture—shared information across individuals. Along with it, another degree of freedom has been added to the extended phenotype, yet one still partially coupled to and having arisen out of genetic evolution.

• *Mimetic–ideational*. When modern humans evolved a capacity for mental representations, the ideational simulation of behavior could commence. The person could now test out mental representations of behavioral trials more rapidly, imagine consequences, and even generate new behavioral mutations (potential innovations) of those trials privately (or cognitively). A new form of trial-and-error learning came into existence with this evolutionary level—one in which our ideas could die in our place (Popper & Eccles, 1977). That evaluative process discards ideas that are likely to fail and retains those more likely to succeed. Eventually, the idea or plan must be tried out in the real world of human action, but its initial development occurs privately as mental representations posing little immediate risk to the individual's survival and welfare. This allows humans to adapt their behavior to the environment and its changes far faster than can occur just by a vicarious learner—indeed, far faster than any known species. The Skinnerian learner has to learn by doing. The vicarious learner has to wait for some innovation in trial-and-error learning to occur before it can be plagiarized by the imitator. The human ideational learner can mentally simulate trials and errors and even mutate representations and behavioral plans to generate more grist for mental evolution. Human *mental* trial-and-error simulation (innovation or creativity) both at the ideational and symbolic levels has created an opportunity for exceptionally rapid adaptation to environmental changes and problems that exceeds any other species. It has also added yet more degrees of freedom to human behavior beyond that of vicarious learners, yet ones still partially coupled to the genetic level that gave rise to the PFC and all of these psychological capacities.

• *Gestural communication.* It has been argued that an early form of communication in humans in their history of evolution was initially gestural (Donald, 1991). This form of communication through movement was believed to be founded on the mimetic–ideational level above in which individuals use mental images to repeatedly initiate behaviors for the sake of rehearsal and improvement. Through such overt rehearsals, others who are watching them might have some understanding of what the individual is attempting to practice and why they are practicing it; this gives rise to gestures as one means of communication. Both the rehearser and observer can understand what is being communicated. In modern humans, such gestural communication is often retained despite loss of symbolic/linguistic communication (aphasias), such as following a stroke or head injury; this suggests that it arises from different mental mechanisms and neurological networks than those that permit language.

• *Symbolic–linguistic.* The evolution of language and the rule-guided behavior it permits is another level of informational evolution that buttresses and even supplants the transmission of information across individuals by observational learning. One therefore finds a human phenotype that can even more rapidly adapt its behavior to the environment, a large part of which is social. It is the existence of the social environment and its rapid changes that likely led to the need (selection pressure) for the development of the observational, communicative (gestural and linguistic), and mental/cognitive (ideational and symbolic) levels of evolution (Barkley, 1997b, 2001).

• *Cultural–artifactual.* The invention of external storage devices for information acquired through language, ideation, and observation permits another level of culture—the sharing of previously acquired knowledge and inventions. These archival artifacts (records, products, objects, tools, etc.) can be transmitted horizontally to others and vertically across subsequent generations. Using the ever-evolving culture, each new generation has the opportunity to reach a higher quality of life and adaptive success than was possible for the previous generation. In its entirety, culture is shared behavioral, gestural, symbolic/linguistic, and recorded information. Even its recorded format evolves and provides yet again another degree of freedom from the level of genetic evolution, despite the fact that *the capacity* for culture arose out of genetic variation (Dennett, 1995, 2003).

The environmental scaffolding provided by culture is itself highly dynamic and its own form of evolution. Current culture is the beneficiary of earlier levels of cultural scaffolding on which it now perches. When studied in detail, the evolution of cultural information proceeds by small stages and steps (ratcheting) (Dawkins, 1987, 1996; Dennett, 1995). This is self-evident in any review of the historical stages of any cultural device or practice, such as the building of cars, planes, and the like, and even that of the principles adopted for organizing entire societies, such as civil and property rights. Laid out in historical sequence, the gradual evolution of a device (actually, information represented by such devices), method, or principle is unmistakable. Over time, huge changes appear to arise from prior gradual improvements (retained useful mutations).

Understanding these multiple levels of universal Darwinism or natural selection is important because the case will be made in later chapters that at least five of these levels arise as a consequence of executive functioning and its components: vicarious learning, ideational, gestural, symbolic–linguistic communication, and cultural.

In Whose Interest Is the Human Extended Phenotype?

It is important to note here that evolution does not proceed for socialistic or collectivist motives but from self-interested ones (Dawkins, 1982).

Situations in which individuals behave solely for the good of others (the group) are unstable because they are prone to invasion by cheaters and free riders who contribute less, or nothing, while benefiting from others' altruistic actions. All cooperative ventures among living organisms exist and are stabilized by the mutual self-interests of the participants and the fact that each derives more benefit from the cooperative venture than they could achieve alone (Dawkins, 1976, 1982; Maynard Smith & Szathmary, 1999; Michod, 1999). That boost in self-benefit from the cooperative venture nearly always involves the eventual division of labor, that is, specialization. The division of labor both boosts self-benefits and binds each to the other in mutual self-support. More can be attained for each through such cooperative activity than either can do alone. This is evident in societal insects as well as at the level of genes combining to form chromosomes, of cells combining to create bodies, and of those bodies behaving cooperatively to form groups. It is self-interest all the way up. That cooperative and apparently altruistic activities may ensue does not alter this contention; it actually serves to explain cooperation's very existence. It will also account for the likely dissolution of cooperative social activities, if conditions change and the individual's self-interests are no longer served by acting cooperatively.

Conclusions

The field of psychology (the study of the behavior of organisms) is a subspecialty of the science of biology (the study of organisms), and this is especially so for the field of neuropsychology (the study of brain–behavior relationships). Evolution is the governing paradigm of biology. It is therefore also a governing paradigm, or should be, in neuropsychology (Barkley, 2001). Major developments in the viewpoints on evolution, such as Dawkins's concepts of selfish genes, his view of extended phenotypes, and the work of many on universal Darwinism are consequently just as applicable to generating hypotheses in neuropsychology as in biology. To neglect or forsake evolution and these concepts is to wall off neuropsychology from its most powerful source of understanding brain–behavior relationships and for generating hypotheses about them.

The next chapter presents an overview of EF, begins to define it more precisely, and moves to apply the concept of an extended phenotype to it.

3

Executive Functioning as an Extended Phenotype

This chapter begins by discussing a more precise definition of EF and how it can be distinguished from non-EF mental functions. It then provides a brief overview of the extended EF phenotype using the general concept from biological evolution (Dawkins, 1982) as discussed in the previous chapter. This chapter concludes with a discussion of the Pre-Executive level of the model. The next four chapters discuss each of the EF levels in more detail as they extend outward from the initial pre-executive phenotype. In discussing the model, the terms "level" and "zone" will be used. This is done with the intent of conveying a hierarchical arrangement of levels as well as zones of influence radiating outward into the ecology of the individual. Each new zone represents effects of the extended phenotype at increasing distances from the genotype and its initial conventional phenotypic zone of expression.

A More Precise Definition of EF

As stipulated toward the end of Chapter 1, I take as my initial starting point the definition of EF as self-regulation (SR). I will show that each component of EF is a specific type of SR—a form of self-directed action aimed at modifying one's behavior so as to make a future goal, end, or outcome more or less likely to occur (Barkley, 1997a, 1997b). EF can therefore be initially defined as *those self-directed actions needed to choose goals and to create, enact, and sustain actions toward those goals*, or more simply as *self-regulation to achieve goals*: EF = SR. Others have made this same connection between the two constructs (Wagner & Heatherton, 2011) and Eslinger (1996), as noted in Chapter 1, found this to be among the most common features of EF in his survey of expert neuropsychologists. Viewing EF as SR offers advantages for both constructs, as others (Hofmann, Friese, Schmeichel, & Baddeley, 2011) acknowledge in discussions of the role of working memory in understanding SR and as discussed in reviews of the linkage of attention networks specifically and EF more generally to self-regulation (Rueda, Posner, & Rothbard, 2011). Since EF is a means for goal-directed action, it is necessary to next define the terms "goals" and "means."

Defining Goals and Means

The literature on the PFC and on EF repeatedly makes reference to their use for goal-directed action (see Sidebar 1.1). Before discussing the means by which humans attain their goals, it helps to briefly define the term "goal" as used in this context. *Goals* are states that result in a decrease in dissatisfaction or unease for an individual relative to the present state (Mises, 1990). Future states that result in a decline in unease (an increase in satisfaction, happiness, or welfare) are states we value; they are desires and wants that we seek to attain, fulfill, and retain (Piekoff, 1993).

The course(s) of action that must be pursued to attain the goal are the *means* to that end.

> A means is what serves to the attainment of any end, goal, or aim. Means are not in the given universe; in this universe there exist only things. A thing becomes a means when human reason employs it for the attainment of some end and human action really employs it for that purpose. Thinking man sees the serviceableness of things, i.e. their ability to minister to ends, and acting man makes them means. It is of primary importance to realize that parts of the external world become means only through the operation of the human mind and its offshoot, human action. External objects are as such only phenomena of the physical universe and the subject matter of the natural sciences. It is human meaning and action which transform them into means. . . . (Mises, 1990, p. 92)

Goals or values are said to have utility—use-value in reducing states of dissatisfaction or unease. There are two types of utility or use-value: *subjective* and *objective* (Mises, 1990). The subjective utility of a goal is strictly personal. It is the degree to which the goal is perceived by that individual to reduce or alleviate that individual's state of dissatisfaction. That degree is its subjective value to that individual. Only that individual, presented with a given context and with any local constraints on choices contained in that situation, can make the determination of utility or value. Only the individual can determine what is "good" to pursue or what is in his or her own longer-term welfare and so compute the subjective use-value of the goal.

The objective utility of a goal is simply the relation between a thing, object, or product and the effect it has the capacity to bring about. Science may permit the means by which to calculate those effects, as in degrees of temperature, units of energy expended (calories), and the like. But this utility or use-value should not be confused with the former subjective one. Humans do not base judgments of value entirely or even partly on the objective use value of a goal or the means to attain it. An action, for example, that raises or lowers the room temperature in my home by adjusting the thermostat by even 3 degrees may be of little or no subjective use value to me but of great current value to my wife even though it is the same objective use value—the action alters room temperature by 3 degrees. Two people given the same information as to the objective use-value of certain means will not necessarily choose the same means or pursue the same ends. That is because no one can judge what another person's subjective state of dissatisfaction is relative to a future state of greater happiness and whether it's worth the pursuit. This makes plain why no individual, collective, or government can or should make decisions concerning "the common good" because there is no such thing as a common good (Mises, 1990). There is only individual good, value, or happiness, and only individuals can decide what that use-value is to them. It is via EF/SR that individuals engage in this process of evaluating ends and means and the subjective use-value of these for their own welfare. To reiterate, it is subjective use-value that drives the goal-directed actions of an individual, not objective use-value. Attempting to understand the choices and actions that individuals make solely by manipulating various parameters of objective use-value will never give a full account of those choices and actions. This means there is a large measure of unpredictability to the choices and actions of others; each individual must take this variability into account in living among and dealing with other people.

An Overview of the EF Extended Phenotype

With the above definitions in mind, the following offers an overview of the EF extended phenotype, which is also summarized in Table 3.1. It is

TABLE 3.1. The Extended Phenotype of EF

Pre-Executive Level

CNS functions
- Routine primary neuropsychological functions, for example, attention, memory, spatial and motor functions, primary emotions and motivations

Behavior
- Automatic activity; operant conditioning

Executive Functioning Levels

Instrumental–Self-Directed Level (internalized mental processes: self-regulation)
- Self-directed attention–self-awareness
- Self-restraint (inhibition)
- Self-directed sensory–motor action (nonverbal working memory; imagination)
- Self-directed private speech (verbal working memory; verbal thought)
- Self-directed appraisal (emotion–motivation)
- Self-directed play (innovation, problem solving)

Methodical–Self-Reliant Level (self-directed actions)
- Use of methods to attain near-term goals
- Self-management across time
- Self-organization and problem solving
- Self-restraint
- Self-motivation
- Self-regulation of emotions
- Social independence, social predation or parasitism, and social self-defense

Tactical–Reciprocal Level (social behaviors)
- Use of tactics—nested sets of methods—to attain midterm goals
- Daily social exchange (sharing, turn-taking, reciprocity, etc.)
- Group living (lower proportion of individual dispersal)
- Beginning of economic behavior (trading)
- Social interdependence (using others to attain goals)

Strategic–Cooperative Level
- Use of strategies—nested sets of tactics—to achieve longer-term goals
- Arrangement of social cooperatives with division of labor
- Acting in unison to achieve common ends and shared benefits
- Origin of larger settlements (further decreases in individual dispersal)
- Stage II: Principled–Mutualistic
  - Use of principles—nested sets of strategies—to achieve long-term goals
  - Pursuit of long-term self-interests by putting others' long-term self-interests ahead of one's own near-term and midterm self-interests
  - Preference for larger delayed over smaller immediate consequences
  - Origin of colonies, cities, city-states, states, and countries

comprised of four levels of EF which emerge from a set of Pre-Executive levels. Each EF level is dealt with in more detail in subsequent chapters.

Pre-Executive Levels

There are at least five levels in the conventional view of a phenotype—the translation of genes into bodies and even behavior. They have been well represented in the conventional model of a phenotype for any given psychological or even physical adaptation or trait. These levels correspond to the genes and their translations into proteins and enzymes that then serve to support brain growth and functioning and the behavior such functioning produces. They can be written as follows:

central nervous system (CNS) relevant genes →
CNS proteins and enzymes → CNS structures →
CNS functions → overt behavior

For the sake of simplicity, I will represent them in my model as being a single set of pre-executive functions as follows, acknowledging that the earlier stages are contained within this expression:

CNS pre-executive functions

At this level, CNS functions and behavior are automatic. The nature of this pre-executive psychological level of the phenotype is discussed later in this chapter, but suffice to say here it is not EF but the prerequisite stage to it.

The Instrumental–Self-Directed Level

Executive functioning first emerges at this level (and zone) of the phenotype. Six of the many psychological functions that exist at the pre-executive level become self-directed to form the initial level of EF. These actions create a conscious mental life for the individual and are as follows: attention—self-awareness, inhibition or self-restraint, self-directed sensory–motor actions (progressing on to mental simulation), self-speech (progressing onward to verbal thought), self-appraisal (evaluation), and self-play. These "actions" may be overt behaviors early in development, but they become self-directed and internalized, thus becoming primarily covert, mental activities later in development. They are forms of self-regulation that work in the service of goal-attainment. An *instrumental*

EF is "instrumental" in that it helps to attain the goal but does not do so by itself. Instrumental EFs are "self-directed" because they are applied only to oneself. Here and for each of the EF/SR levels in this model, the second term in the label used for each indicates its social significance. This level is discussed in detail in Chapter 4. The extended phenotype at this level is as follows:

CNS pre-executive functions → executive (self-regulatory) functions

The Methodical–Self-Reliant Level

This level is concerned with overt goal-directed actions and behavior. A method is a short chain of actions that achieve a given goal much like the steps of a recipe. No single action in the sequence accomplishes the goal, but together, as a sequence, the actions accomplish the goal. Such a goal is often near-term, necessitating short chains of actions to attain it. A method is more complex than a single action or gesture because it is built up from such simpler actions. The methodical level is "self-reliant" because the individual's goals tend to be focused on growing independence from and self-defense against others. It also includes a capacity for social predation—the use of others in a parasitic way for one's own ends that are not mutually beneficial and against which others will employ forms of self-defense. Chapter 5 discusses this level and its zone of effects in more detail. Unique to this level is the concept of executive behavior as distinct from executive cognition. Executive cognition comprises the private mental and self-directed events subjective to the individual, while executive behavior includes the overt and observable activities being driven by those mental representations (executive cognition). As part of this overt self-regulatory behavior, people engage in reconfigurations of the physical environment to assist with or amplify their self-regulation and their goal-directed actions. The extended phenotype can now be written as follows:

CNS pre-executive functions → executive (self-regulatory) functions → executive (self-regulatory) adaptive behavior → self-organization of environmental arrangements (products, artifacts)

The Tactical–Reciprocal Level

This level and the one that follows represent the social symbiotic levels of EF. At the Tactical–Reciprocal level and zone, relationships with others are no longer those of social parasitism/predation and self-defense against others' parasitism; others now become means for attaining goals that are mutually beneficial—socially symbiotic. The term "tactical" is used to mean *sets of methods* clustered together to comprise longer-chain action sequences that achieve a higher order, longer-term goal. Each method within a "tactic" achieves a necessary subgoal. The term "tactical" is also used in its traditional social meaning of an adjustment in one's actions relative to the actions or anticipated actions of others as in a military engagement. However, the tactical level is also associated with initial types of social relationships in which a person uses another in a mutually beneficial way to assist with achievement of personal goals, as in reciprocity, exchange, and mutual sharing. Therefore, this level is also titled "reciprocal." Chapter 6 covers this level. The EF extended phenotype at this level looks as follows:

CNS pre-executive functions → executive (self-regulatory) functions →
executive (self-regulatory) adaptive behavior → self-organization
of environmental arrangements (products, artifacts) → self-organizing
of social arrangements involving symbiotic reciprocal exchanges with others

The Strategic–Cooperative Level

The term "strategic" or *strategy* refers to a set or sets of tactics that are now hierarchically organized into much longer sequences of actions extended over longer time periods to attain much later goals than one was capable of doing at the previous level of the EF extended phenotype. In other words, methods are nested under tactics that are nested under strategies that can eventually attain goals at a considerable distance in time. The second social meaning of "strategic" is also applicable. It refers to a set of social tactics one is using within a larger social network, over a longer time frame than would be seen at the tactical level. The strategic level thus refers to a higher order of social engagement for the purpose of attaining personal goals, such as participating in "cooperative" activities to attain goals that no individual could achieve alone. Here the term "cooperative" does not mean simply going along or getting along with others in its most general sense. It means acting in unison or as a unity with others to achieve goals that cannot be achieved alone or through mere reciprocity (exchange). The individual becomes part of a larger unit or cooperative. Hence the social term "cooperative" is also used for this level. See Chapter 7 for more detail on this level. It can now be expressed as follows:

CNS pre-executive functions → CNS executive (self-regulatory) functions →
executive (self-regulatory) adaptive behavior → self-organization
of environmental arrangements (products, artifacts) → self-organizing
of social arrangements for reciprocal exchanges with others →
social arrangements for cooperative ventures with others

The four previous levels or zones are sufficient to represent the model of an extended EF phenotype for most purposes. Yet I will argue that modern civilizations have reached a point in providing sufficient cultural scaffolding for an additional stage of this last level to be identified in developed societies—it is the Principled–Mutualistic stage representing the broadest social ecology or context in which many, though by no means all, individuals currently live. A principle is a set or sets of strategies that are being employed to achieve the longest range, most complex, and most abstract forms of human goal-seeking. It refers to principled behavior. It is also "mutualistic" to reflect the individual's use of a much larger and longer-term group-living arrangement (a community) of individuals. Each individual strives to look out for others' long-term self-interests, provided those others do the same. It is volitional, freely chosen mutual aid as in a symbiotic relationship (mutually beneficial).

The extended phenotype can now be written as follows:

CNS pre-executive functions → CNS executive (self-regulatory) functions →
executive (self-regulatory) adaptive behavior → self-organization
of environmental arrangements (products, artifacts) → self-organizing
of social arrangements for reciprocal exchanges with others →
social arrangements for cooperative ventures with others →
social arrangements for mutualistic communities

I argue that each new level comes into existence because of an increase in the PFC's developmental capacities, particularly that capacity involved in contemplating the future. These capacities are discussed next. The maturational course they require to reach full expression likely spans three decades, the time it may take for the PFC—and the EF system that depends on it—to reach full maturity. The essential point throughout the model is that the ultimate purposes of the EF/SR system are inherently social. Moreover, individuals do not employ the highest levels of EF under all circumstances with all other people. They exercise judgment in specific contexts in deciding at what level of the EF hierarchy they will engage in interactions and transactions with another person. Some people they avoid, and they may use levels of self-defense that arise at the Methodical–Self-Reliant level. For others, they may engage in reciprocity, while for others they may choose to engage in cooperative or even mutualistic ventures. Individuals range across these levels on any given day in any particular context as they interact with various individuals.

Eight Emerging Developmental Capacities Arising from EF

Attempts to describe the functions of the frontal lobe within the framework of a single characteristic unitary defect appear to be doomed to failure from the outset, because the frontal lobe is no small ganglia, no tiny knot of tissue, but a vast corpus the functions of which in all probability are as numerous as the frontal lobes are large. Although we may seek no one basic defect associated with damage to the frontal lobes, that does not preclude the search for broad principles of action upon which the functioning of the frontal lobes may be based. (Dimond, 1980, pp. 508–509)

I concur. The complexity of the PFC, of necessity, will be matched by the complexity of EF which it supports. Research on the functions of and damage to the PFC briefly summarized in Chapter 1 give rise to the possibility that these functions may be usefully classified along eight developmental neurocognitive dimensions. At each level in the model of EF, these eight developmental parameters change with maturation of the PFC and drive the outward extension of the EF phenotype into daily human personal, social, community, and culture activities. They can be thought of as emerging neuropsychological capacities that influence human actions, especially those beyond the automatic, Pre-Executive level. While I distinguish them here, they should be viewed as highly interrelated and as a totality when the EF system reaches full adult maturation. These capacities can be used to help distinguish between the levels even though the boundaries between the levels should be considered soft or fuzzy given the dimensional rather than categorical nature of these capacities.

Spatial Capacity

This refers to the spatial distance over which the individual is contemplating a goal and the necessary means to attain it. It can be indexed by identifying the increasing outward spread of the effects of self-directed actions. From their initial range at proximal space, they spread into more distant destinations in physical (and eventually social) environments. One effect of this cognitive capacity (by which it can be indexed) is that individuals come to purposefully rearrange or organize their surrounding physical environment to assist in goal attainment—a radius of environmental self-organization that grows in scope with development.

Temporal Capacity

This reflects how far into the future the individual is capable of contemplating a goal. Also called a time horizon, it is evident in the span of time between a likely future event (i.e., a deadline) and the individual beginning to prepare for the event. Metaphorically, it reflects a mental window on time that opens increasingly wider with maturation of the PFC. Initially it comprises only minutes, then hours, then days, weeks, and finally months and years. It is apparently localized to the right prefrontal lobe, although assisted by networks connecting this region to the basal ganglia and the cerebellum (Picton, Stuss, Shallice, Alexander, & Gillingham, 2006; Wheeler, Stuss, & Tulving, 1997). It is highly likely to be related to spatial capacity because taking actions across geographical distances (space) also requires time. A capacity for reckoning the time needed to traverse space and attain the goal will be important in actions across spatial distances. Eventually, so will be a sense of timing and timeliness of such actions.

Motivational Capacity

This arises out of the previous two capacities, especially the temporal one. It can be distinguished by the fact that this capacity reflects a "hot" appraisal of that future, while the spatial and temporal capacities above are comprised of "cold" cognitive parameters or purely information. It can be thought of as a motivational time horizon as it reflects the personal valuation of a delayed consequence, future goal, or outcome that the individual is contemplating. It is often evident in complex emotional–motivational–arousal responses (feelings) of individuals concerning the goals they are contemplating. The more highly valued or preferred the consequences, the more willing individuals are to increase the time delay and the spatial distances needed to attain that goal. The temporal aspect of this motivational parameter is represented in the concept from behavior analysis of temporal or reward discounting—the fact that individuals increasingly discount the value of a consequence by the degree of time delay for that consequence. However, across development, humans manifest an increase in the valuation of delayed consequences or a more gradual decline in the slope of this function (Green, Fry, & Myerson, 1994; Green, Myerson, Lichtman, Rosen, & Fry, 1996). It is identical to the economic concept known as time preference (Mises, 1990) and can be usefully considered as a gradient representing delay of gratification (Mischel, 1983; Mischel & Ayduk, 2011; Mischel, Shoda, & Peake, 1989). Noteworthy, however, is that there is also likely to be a spatial equivalent to such a temporal discounting function, which itself may interact with the temporal one, as when goals that occur at increasing distances from the individual require not just additional effort to attain but also additional time to get there.

Inhibitory Capacity

This concerns the extent to which and the duration over which individuals must inhibit their responses to prepotent events, restrain their actions, and otherwise subordinate their immediate interests for the sake of the goal. Eventually such actions will also come to be subordinated to any interests of others with whom the individual is attempting to reciprocate or cooperate to attain a goal. This capacity interacts with the previous capacities as is evident in the fact that individuals with a high time preference or those who steeply discount the value of delayed consequences are frequently described as or identified as impulsive, selfish, and even irrational (Rachlin & Ranieri, 1992) and as having an inability to delay gratification (Mischel, 1983; Mischel & Ayduk, 2011).

Conceptual/Abstract Capacity

This reflects the degree of abstractness of any rules that are being considered and followed to attain the goal. It ranges from the most simple, specific, and concrete level of rules to the most abstract, general, conceptual, and complex principles. It can be illustrated by contrasting simple self-directed rules, such as "stop" or "wait" to highly conceptual rules such as "do unto others as you would have them do unto you" or one that states that "all individuals should be presumed innocent until proven guilty."

Behavioral–Structural Capacity

This is essentially the motor consequences of the other dimensions and indicates the degree of behavioral complexity and hierarchical structuring of the actions needed to bridge the time period and distance between the moment and the contemplated goal. It is a capacity for structuring increasingly complex, hierarchically organized, and appropriately sequenced actions toward goals. That complexity is evident in the number and levels of nested sets of actions that will need to be planned, sequenced, and then performed, as well as the timing of those actions to effectively attain the anticipated goal being contemplated. It is represented in this model by the first term in the label of each EF level—instrumental, methodical, tactical, strategic, and even principled. This capacity is also evident in the hierarchical organization of the PFC on which such functioning is based (Badre, 2008; Botvinich, 2008).

Social Capacity

This refers to the number of other individuals (and eventually social networks) with which the individual must interact, reciprocate, and cooperate so as to effectively attain the goal being contemplated. Of course, it would include the length of time and complexity involved in the interactions required with each person.

Cultural Capacity

This last capacity refers to the degree of cultural information and devices (methods, inventions, products, etc.) or *scaffolding* that the individual is adopting to attain the goal under contemplation. Culture is shared information (Durham, 1991; Janicki & Krebs, 1998; Symons, 1992; Tooby & Cosmides, 1992) inherited from prior generations and created and shared within the current one. The origins of culture in human evolution are of little concern here other than the fact that humans create and use such shared information to their own advantage, either as means to ends (e.g., computers for writing) or as ends in themselves (e.g., the pleasure of appreciating music and art). Various models of the evolution of culture exist (see the excellent review by Janicki & Krebs, 1998), some of which emphasize culture as arising out of biological evolution while others argue that it is a second form of inheritance (universal Darwinism) that may be partially or entirely decoupled from genetic evolution as described in Chapter 2. While I favor the latter (see, e.g., Durham, 1997), the question of which model is correct is immaterial to the argument here. What matters is that the individual is going to use the EF system to capitalize on the available shared information as a means to attaining goals and improving long-term welfare. I share the view that cultural information is not passively received or absorbed by the brain;

it is actively adopted by individuals to achieve their goals (Janicki & Krebs, 1998; Tooby & Cosmides, 1992). Culture requires a brain that is prepared to both receive it and create it. Indeed Taylor (2010) has argued that this reciprocal interplay of human ancestors with available technology was a major driving force in the evolution of modern humans. Absent the availability of cultural inventions, a goal may not be able to be accomplished or even contemplated. Conversely, absent the brain mechanisms needed to adopt culture (the EF system), such information is of no use to the individual. EF is viewed here as a set of components installed in the human extended phenotype by biological evolution. It creates a mind already receptive to culture and to using cultural devices as a means to the individual's own ends. Cultural information may well serve to boost EF capacity and provides much of the content on which the EF system is working. But EF is not purely a result of culture or learning; it is a universal human trait. Eventually individuals give back to the culture through their own inventions and discoveries, making the relationship between individual and culture bidirectional (Tooby & Cosmides, 1992). The preexisting culture that a human may be born into can ratchet upward and outward the extended phenotypic zones in which they may be capable of participating at maturation and greatly extend the effects of their phenotype at distances that were not possible for earlier generations or for themselves at an earlier age. Advances in telecommunication technology such as from telegraphs to telephones, to cell phones, and now to the Internet and other social network devices are but a few examples of how cultural scaffolding can provide opportunities for phenotypic effects at distances impossible for previous generations of humans. Advances in cultural devices (technology) can also permit people to off-load some of the storage and effort used in EF to external devices, making goal attainment easier and inventing new goals not previously possible. Also, advances in formal social organizations, such as laws, constitutions, and forms of government, can serve to ratchet up an individual to a higher level of extended EF phenotypic functioning not permitted to either earlier generations or those born into less advanced societies. Both illustrate the increasing role that preexisting and newly invented cultural means or scaffolding play as one moves up these levels of the extended EF phenotype.

There is no question that children must undergo extensive training in cultural knowledge, practices, and devices (scaffolding) by parents and teachers. The longer a culture exists, the more "scaffolding" it has available to provide to children. This information concerning its practices, procedures, products, and other information can serve as means to ends, and even ends themselves, within the society. Education can be usefully portrayed as the construction of this type of cognitive and social scaffolding via the active training involved in pedagogy. This training is not merely the passive display of cultural information to the child recipient. It is active training in its content, meaning, and use. And it is the active pursuit of such training by the recipient as well. This training creates the cultural scaffolding on which the child's EF system can capitalize in pursuit of goals and ratchets up both the means that one can use to pursue such goals and even the goals that can be pursued. Availability of and training in the cultural knowledge base is an essential part of this developmental dimension. In modern societies, this scaffolding is extensive and often must be acquired through sequential stages, such as through instruction in arithmetic, algebra, and calculus as well as geometry and trigonometry, and it often requires years or even a decade or more to complete its formal stage.

The first three capacities above—spatial, temporal, and motivational—are likely the most fundamental to the development of EF. They generate the capacity for a sense of the self, a sense of one's current state, and a conscious sense of the hypothetical future—an ability to imagine goals ever more distant in time and space and to contemplate the action plans needed to attain them. Each level and zone of the EF extended phenotype will be characterized along these eight developmental dimensions starting with the Pre-Executive level covered later in this chapter.

Vicarious Learning and Innovation as Parts of EF's Extended Phenotype

Having mentioned the developmental capacity for adopting culture above, let us now consider how this capacity may have arisen in evolution. It is typically thought to be based on the human abilities for vicarious learning and for innovation; both arise from EF at the Instrumental–Self-Directed level. Recall from Chapter 2 that humans possess an unusual adaptation—vicarious or observational learning. It involves not only immediate and delayed imitation of the actions of others but also the immediate and delayed suppression of behavior through observation of the failures and adversities of others. Observational learning provides a human with a form of experiential theft or, more accurately, plagiarism. An individual can simply witness the performance of another human and immediately re-imagine that performance. That revisualization allows a person to readjust his or her own behavior accordingly. This

adjustment can result in copying the actions of another if it was successful. Or it can result in subsequently suppressing that failed response of
another in the observer's own repertoire. By this means, at least initially,
humans develop a protoculture. Culture is essentially the spreading of
information across individuals, in this case a behavior pattern. Information spreads across individuals simply from their witnessing the experiences (means and goals, products and outcomes) of others. That spreading effect can sweep through a small social group or through an entire
population of vicarious learners. Language clearly complements and
amplifies this type of learning and so creates a more complex form of
culture based on it. But even that more complex form of culture requires
the more fundamental faculty of vicarious learning, given that learning
from language is likely built on the earlier level of vicarious learning and
mimetic (gestural) communication (Donald, 1991, 1993).

Consider as well that humans are also highly innovative; this is
another component of EF to be discussed in the Instrumental–Self-
Directed level (see Chapter 4). We use this component of EF to engage
in private forms of trial-and-error learning—mental simulations of our
behavior and of various combinations of such behavior. When combined
with vicarious learning, it is therefore possible for an individual living in
one geographic locality, say Boston, Massachusetts, in the United States,
to discover through mental trial-and-error learning (i.e., cognitive simulations or thinking) an entirely new, more efficient, and more effective
means of achieving some widely desired human goal. By others observing this activity, the innovation then spreads rapidly and exponentially
through the surrounding population. This results in an ever-widening
rippling effect of the behavioral actions of one person on those of others
to an extent that over a matter of hours, days, or weeks this habit pattern
now influences a sizeable percentage of the population. And it does so at
a geographic distance that may reach people living on the opposite coast
of the country, such as Los Angeles, California. From there, the effect
can spread internationally.

Yet we must also recognize that the original creator of this invention was likely relying on cultural information, products, and other artifacts in the act of recombination and innovation, having used vicarious
learning and language to acquire such information. This illustrates the
bidirectional pathways between the individual creating culture and also
adopting and utilizing it for adaptive success and innovation.

These human EF capacities for mental innovation and vicarious
learning produce effects at both a spatial and temporal distance that is
stunning in their breadth and scope. They account for a large part of

human cultural practices and their cultural evolution apart from genetic evolution. To count as part of an extended phenotype, recall from Chapter 2 that such effects must not be mere by-products but must alter the success, wealth, social status, mating opportunities, or longevity of the individual (and his or her kin) who initiated the discovery (and of those who adopted it). At the specific distance from the genotype where such feedback no longer exists, the effect is not an extended phenotypic one. How can such feedback occur at such geographic distances as cited above in the example of vicarious learning and cultural invention? It occurs through trade and the monetary economy associated with it. To the extent that the inventor derives any benefits from the adoption of the invention by others at a distance, a mechanism for such feedback exists and thereby boosts the wealth (resources) of the individual and hence his or her survival and reproductive success. Language, as a proxy for vicariously learning, can further facilitate and amplify the breadth and rapidity of this outwardly spreading influence. There is the potential for dramatic and widespread effects of an individual's EF phenotype on that of others at great spatial and temporal distances; those effects can then feed back to affect adaptive and reproductive success (or failure) of the innovative individual.

Human vicarious learning and language are part of the extended human EF phenotype because natural selection acts to increase or decrease the individual's survival and reproduction at any of the extended phenotypic levels, not merely those closest to the skin (the endophenotype). Moreover, the impact of vicarious learning and mental innovation does not just benefit others who copy or adopt the means or products of the inventor. They also provide the individual inventor with self-regulation and subsequent self-improvement. Those benefits cannot be overstated; these mental faculties result in a speed and breadth of behavioral development and improvement both within and between individuals unrivaled in any other species. They also form the principal basis of human pedagogy and culture.

The Pre-Executive Levels and Zones

As in some previous models of EF processes (Fuster, 1997; Stuss & Benson, 1986), a level of human brain functioning and associated sensory–motor actions or behavior exists that is not considered executive. Why they are not considered to be "executive" has not always been made very clear, as discussed in Chapter 1, though it will become so later in this section. This basic level arises from non-prefrontal brain structures and their functions and mainly arise from the posterior cortical and basal zones. It also includes the functions related to motor preparation and execution as they arise in motor regions of the frontal cortex (sensory–motor strip, primary, secondary, and tertiary motor zones). The assignment of functions and behavior to particular neurological structures, networks, and their electrochemical functions is not of concern here and is unnecessary to building a model of EF at the psychological level of analysis. Consequently, brain structure and neuronal functioning receive little further attention here.

Included at the Pre-Executive level of the model are many of the routine neuropsychological functions such as attention, alertness, visual–spatial performance, autonomic–emotional actions, memory, sensory–perceptual functions, language, and motor abilities (see Stuss & Benson, 1986). These brain functions are responsible for the stimulus–response, moment-to-moment, and largely unconscious or automatic activities of the organism as it goes about sustaining its life in its natural habitat. This level can be fruitfully regarded as the "automatic" level of human activity often described in models of self-regulation (Kahneman, 2011), such as in feedback loop theory (Carver & Scheier, 2011), Gross's emotional self-regulation model (Gross, 2007; Ochsner & Gross, 2005, 2008), attention control models (Rueda, Posner, & Rothbard, 2011), and the concept of effortful control (Eisenberg, Smith, & Spinrad, 2011), among others.

As Gross (2007) has described it, this level likely consists of four stages in a sequence represented as

situation → attention → appraisal → response

If amended to include the consequences of responses that then serve as feedback and so affect the subsequent probability of this sequence, it represents operant conditioning. These stages of processing usually occur in rapid succession and outside of self-awareness or self-consciousness, which come later at the executive level of the model. This pre-executive pathway is concerned with more immediate or near-term concrete goals and with attaining primitive motivational and appetitive values (goals) that contribute to the individual's short-term welfare, as is often the case in other primates. It gives rise to species-specific behavior patterns as is evident in many animals. It also includes the second level of evolution (universal Darwinism) discussed in Chapter 2, that being Skinnerian (operantly conditioned) behavior which has the structure of stimulus–

response–consequence. Primary emotions occur at this automatic level. They may be signals to individuals that alert them to situations that have been unconsciously appraised as affecting their near-term well-being, as Darwin proposed (see Leary & Guadagno, 2011). They may therefore serve as an attention-heightening and redirecting influence. But none of this is considered to be executive.

Such pre-executive functions are important to consider given the assertion below that some of them are used in the creation of the initial EF level (the Instrumental–Self-Directed level) and the initiation and maintenance of short-term goal-directed actions that next level creates. What distinguishes these pre-executive functions from those at the next EF level is that they (1) do not arise as a consequence of conscious, volitional, and effortful self-directed actions by the individual; and (2) are not consciously future or goal-directed, purposive, or intentional in their typical activities. They are directed at the temporal "now" and the proximal space in the ecology of the organism. They are not in and of themselves forms of self-regulation and are therefore not components of EF.

At this Pre-Executive level, we can characterize the eight developmental capacities, introduced earlier, as follows. The *spatial* distance over which the individual is pursuing goals is quite proximal to them; that is because there is little or no contemplation of this parameter. The degree to which the individual is reorganizing and producing effects on their spatial environment to assist with self-regulation is nonexistent. The *temporal* distance or time horizon they are consciously employing, if they are conscious of it at all, is very near and characterized as "the now." Behavior is being focused on moment-to-moment survival. The *motivational* horizon is therefore very near. In economic terms the time preference is very high; temporal discounting is quite steep. The individual's behavior is focused on those goals, rewards, or consequences that are very proximal in time. The degree of *inhibition* or self-restraint available at this level and required for attaining proximal goals is minimal. The *behavioral* complexity needed to achieve those outcomes is rather simple and so of relatively short duration and of little complexity (the number of nested sets of subgoal means and ends that must be combined to attain the goal is minimal or nonexistent). The level of *conceptualization or abstractness* of the rules that are being used to pursue a goal is nonexistent. Indeed, symbolism and language could not arise in such an organism. The *social* involvement and complexity being used to pursue goals is minimal or nonexistent. The conscious planning and use of social reciprocity and cooperative behavior would not be possible at this level. Where such behavior may exist in other organisms, it has arisen through the genetic level of evolution and not through conscious choice. The purposeful inclusion of others in efforts to attain a goal is largely unnecessary. The fact that other people may provide assistance to the individual is not a result of any plan by that individual to include those others. Its provision is more a function of the concerns of other individuals about this person and their perception of the person's needs for such assistance in order to survive. The cultural scaffolding being utilized here is also limited or nonexistent and arises only in the fact that prior cultural information and artifacts may exist in the environment that the individual happens to encounter. But the individual could not absorb them or use them and so is not likely to be purposefully or intentionally drawing on such products to attain their goals.

This is a primitive, unthinking, unreasoning, un-self-regulating level of existence. If this were the only zone possessed by humans, we would likely cease to exist in our current form; we possess few other adaptations to assist with our survival in competition with other species. But this level does serve as the initial basis for the evolution of EF in humans and in the development of the individual's EF. It will eventually be governed by the EF system in the service of goal-directed activities.

4

The Instrumental–
Self-Directed Level

EF arises at the Instrumental–Self-Directed level of the human extended phenotype. This level likely incorporates those components of EF identified in current cognitive views of EF and its measurement. However, those components as described in the present model take on an entirely new character as will become evident below. These are the EFs that are most proximal to and arise from moment-to-moment PFC activity. While they can be localized to various PFC regions and networks, it is not necessary to do so for the validity of the model. This level is not some passive exercise in conveying information through modules of some processing system as some information-processing models of EF have portrayed it. It represents active, effortful, largely conscious human actions-to-the-self, often called controlled or System 2 activities (Kahneman, 2011). Applying the concept of the extended phenotype to this level, we can represent it as:

CNS pre-executive functions → CNS executive (self-directed) functions

There are six self-directed actions (EF components or functions) in which humans engage at this level: attention, inhibition, sensory–motor action, speech, appraisal (emotion and motivation), and play. Each of these EF components arises via the same developmental sequence and process. That sequence is best illustrated by the *self-direction* and *internalization* of speech described by Vygotsky (1962, 1978, 1987; see also Diaz & Berk, 1992). These two processes—self-direction and internalization—cause this Instrumental EF level to come into existence from the pre-executive one. They give the human mind and human language some of their unique properties (Bronowski, 1977). Each EF component at this level is a form of action (behavior) that was initially outer-directed—that is, directed toward sensing and responding to the environment at the Pre-Executive level. Each eventually becomes self-directed during child development as a means to alter subsequent behavior from what it would have otherwise been. Each serves to manage or modify the individual's ongoing behavior and to mediate or bridge the delay to the consequence itself. Talking to yourself, counting to yourself, or visualizing task-relevant images to yourself are all self-directed means young children use to attempt to successfully mediate delays to later consequences (goals) and are therefore more likely to obtain those consequences (Mischel, 1983; Mischel et al., 1989). This *self-direction* of action is being done so as to increase the likelihood of attaining a goal or end state. That is the tripartite definition of self-regulation (SR), which states that SR is (1) an action directed at the self, (2) so as to modify a subsequent behavior from what it would otherwise have been, (3) so as to alter the likelihood of a delayed consequence (goal).

The second key process is *internalization*. Over the course of human development the self-directed sensory–motor actions (and later, self-speech) being used for self-regulation undergo internalization—they become private or "cognitive" in form. This is done by the suppression of the musculoskeletal movements that comprise these actions. This permits the brain functions that give rise to them to continue unabated while the peripheral expressions of those brain actions are being largely inhibited from public display. The brain activities that give rise to the initially publicly observable self-directed action are prevented from being released into the spinal column for execution and thus remain in the brain. A private form of self-directed activities arises and probably represents the conscious mind. This prevention of externally executed behavior most likely involves an inhibitory switching mechanism probably in the basal ganglia and associated neural networks (see Saint-Cyr, 2003) that serve to suppress the execution of motor actions during cortical preparations to act. The process of privatization grants the individual a capacity to generate actions in the brain (mind) without acting them out in the environment and thus forms a type of simulation of behavioral trials. Perhaps it also explains why disruption of the basal ganglia, as in Tourette syndrome, results in an involuntary release of cortically activated motor and verbal behavior that is inappropriate to the context.

Regardless of the neurological mechanism responsible for privatization (an interesting research question in its own right), it creates a conscious mental life for the individual; one based on private sensory–motor and linguistic activities. The individual possesses a set of six mind tools that can be used privately or cognitively for mentally simulating reality and their potential actions within it. Mental simulations are imaginary constructions that can be used to contemplate and mentally test out various rearrangements of the material world and one's own behavior within it. These activities comprise what is meant by the term "executive functioning" at this level.

EF in Six Self-Directed Acts

Each of the six self-regulatory actions elaborated here is a conscious, voluntary, effortful action.

Self-Directed Attention–Self-Awareness

Self-awareness is vital as the starting point for EF. It has been acknowledged so in prior reviews of PFC functions as the pinnacle EF or central executive and may arise out of more than just self-directed sensing. The self-direction of attention comes to create self-awareness. Logic alone requires that it precede the existence of the other EF components as they all presuppose a sense of self. One cannot direct an action back on the self for self-regulation if one has no sense of self. It must be the first to arise in development and may well be the most important as it serves as a precursor to all other forms of self-regulation. It is here that the individual becomes conscious or aware of the entirety of their internal and external states, drives, wants, and actions and so achieves an organized, integrated unity or sense of self.

Self-Restraint (Executive Inhibition)

The second EF component in importance must be self-restraint or executive inhibition. This is so because no further egoistic actions can occur until the individual ceases directing action toward the environment, however briefly. One cannot respond to the environment with action and self-direct an action simultaneously. This type of inhibition achieves a *separation* of the external event from the eventual sensory–motor responses that will be enacted in response to it. This creates a decoupling of the stimulus from its response that was typical of the earlier, automatic form of behavior that is so well studied in operant conditioning. The capacity to delay action likely co-develops with the capacity to prolong the sensory impression of the stimulus (see below) as neurons for both appear to sit adjacent to each other in the PFC (Goldman-Rakic, 1995). This separation or decoupling requires inhibition of the prepotent motor response that such sensory events typically generate at the automatic level of brain functioning. This appears to be largely localized to the frontal-striatal circuitry and an indirect routing aspect of the basal ganglia (Saint-Cyr, 2003). It would also require inhibition of attention to unrelated events and their sensory impressions (a resistance to distraction) at the time the primary sensory representation is being prolonged or re-imagined.

This EF component represents self-stopping, or the ability to interrupt the flow of more automatic ongoing behavior. It involves three quasi-distinct forms: (1) the capacity to suppress or otherwise disrupt or prevent the execution of a prepotent or dominant response to an event (the response that has been previously associated with reinforcement or has the highest likelihood of being performed under ordinary circumstances); (2) the capacity to interrupt an ongoing sequence of behavior toward a goal if it is proving to be ineffective; and (3) the capacity to protect the self-directed actions that will subsequently occur and the goal-directed actions they are guiding from interference by external and internal goal-irrelevant events (creating a freedom from distraction or a resistance to interference).

For goal-directed behavior to arise, attention must be shifted away from the moment and external reality and turned toward the self and the mentally contemplated future for that self—the goal. The temporal gap created by the deferred response provides the opportunity for further self-regulatory actions and the eventual goal-directed behavior they will actually initiate.

Self-Directed Sensory–Motor Action

Self-directed sensory–motor action is an alternative means of describing what others may call a nonverbal working memory system. I prefer to understand it in Vygotsky-like terms as a type of self-directed human action. In this case, it is largely the use of self-directed vision that is visual imagery. A person literally re-sees images, typically engaging the right dorsolateral prefrontal cortex as well as the posterior visual association areas (D'Esposito et al., 1995, 1997). This is not just done with vision but with all of the senses, such as re-hearing, re-smelling, and re-feeling. Done jointly, the mental representation can consist of more than just an image alone but a fully integrated sensory representation. What this self-directed sensory activity serves to do is to prolong the referent, that is, the environmental stimulus or event that has triggered the initial or primary sensory perception. Doing so may not be necessary as long as the stimulus or event remains present in the sensory fields. As long as it does so, it continues to trigger the sensory perception of it. Prolongation can be exceptionally beneficial when the stimulus or event disappears in the external world or is no longer able to be perceived (it may have gone behind something). That is because the individual can now have a sense that the object or stimulus may have continued to exist even though it is no longer perceptible. You will recognize this capacity for prolongation of sensory representations in their absence in the external world as the basis for the development of object permanence in infants. Predators and enemies can hide, and any mental function that can give rise to an understanding that the object continues to exist despite its disappearance from the sensory receptors would be incredibly advantageous to survival, even more so if that predator or competitor is a conspecific—another human.

The prolongation of environmental referents can now result in their being stored as distinct memories, such that the individual cannot just prolong the referent after its disappearance in reality, but store a representation of that prolonged referent for later retrieval. This is probably the basis for episodic memory, or a recollection of a personally perceived event that occurs within a specific temporal context or sequence. Recalling such episodic memories can eventually come to trigger the motor responses that typically occur in the presence of the actual environmental event. By prolonging, storing, and re-presenting the initial stimulus in mental form, the individual can now re-imagine the stimulus and hence re-trigger the associated response to it. The person can now use this re-imagining of past sensory–motor events to self-elicit action in the absence of the primary stimulus typically eliciting it. This permits the person to reenact the behavior repeatedly. Behavioral reenactments, or mimesis, being triggered by mental re-presentations of sensory stimuli can become means of practice and rehearsal. They can become means to further perfect the response to the actual environmental event the next time it appears in that external world. This initial rehearsal is publicly observable, yet it is incredibly advantageous for improving subsequent behavior. Humans often demonstrate public rehearsals of actions they intend to use later under real circumstances. When this behavioral rehearsal becomes internalized, it is a means for the private simulation of human actions and may be the basis for human rituals (Rossano,

2011). This internalization of sensory–motor actions also explains the importance of the cerebellum in EF or "higher cognition" (Diamond, 2000; Houk & Wise, 1995). Given its importance for the execution of public behavior, it would be just as essential for its private simulation.

Once this rehearsal to the self has become privatized or internalized by the mechanism of internalization noted earlier, it can now bequeath to the individual a private means of reenactment, practice, or rehearsal. Now, both the initial sensory representations and the motor actions they trigger can be executed covertly, or in the mind. This imaginary construction serves as a template for the imaginary repetition of a behavior for purposes of practice. This, I believe, becomes the source of the human capacity for the imaginary construction of a hypothetical reality and of our actions within it. Such images and larger imaginary structures are ideas. This is therefore the EF component that gave rise to a form of ideational evolution discussed in Chapter 2. This capacity for private mental evolution of ideas would have given humans a more rapid means of adapting to their environment—the gift of mental simulation. While this may well be the basis for what other neuropsychologists have called working memory, that term hardly does justice to the process that reframing it as self-directed actions can provide. Some research suggests that such "working memory" may be the function that provides the foundation for some of the other EF components, such as the mental manipulation of information and problem solving (McCabe et al., 2010).

As will be discussed below, this component is probably the origin of human hindsight (revisualizing past reality and one's actions), foresight (imagining a future goal and the actions needed to attain it), and awareness of self across time. Every goal represents a want, a desire, a value, or more generally a change in the current state of wants and needs (a reduction in dissatisfaction; an increase in well-being or satisfaction). Juxtaposing a goal against a current state represents a conflict between the current state of individuals (what they feel now) and what the individuals desire it to be (what they want that state to be). The conflict is, by definition, a problem for the individual. To be able to address such conflicts, the individuals must be aware of them; they must be *self-conscious* of these current and future inner states. Moreover, the foresight the individual is going to employ is largely one of self-interest across time—the future usually being contemplated is one's own future. One must be aware not only of the current inner state, but of what is possible to change or achieve—the desired future state for one's self. Thus, there must not only be a capacity for self-awareness, but this capacity must include a temporal component (self-now vs. self-future)—*awareness of self across time*. This has been called autonoetic awareness and is attributed to the PFC, especially in the right hemisphere (Wheeler et al., 1997). Humans are time-binding animals, binding the future to the present, as Fuster (1997) noted concerning cross-temporal structures of events, responses, and their likely outcomes that are a major function of the PFC. Self-directed sensory–motor action is hypothesized to be the EF component that achieves that time-binding function.

The capacity to imagine a hypothetical future from an experienced past is one of the three most important or foundational EFs. The other two are self-directed attention (self-awareness) and self-restraint as noted above. Together they create the human sense of the future. Important to notice here is that the future being conceived is not the entire future for all or even for this individual—it is a fractional future. The individual is contemplating what may happen relative to a given context and set of actions being considered at that time in order to attain a specific goal. Moreover, the fractional future under consideration is not just the probable future of what is likely to come to pass if conditions remain as they are, though that is an important function in its own right. It is also the capacity to conceive of a possible future—what might be rather than just what is. Humans can conceive of a possible future and thereby have an opportunity to change the course of their actions from what it would otherwise have been; they can change the likely future.

The first three EF components—self-awareness, self-restraint (inhibition), and self-directed sensory–motor actions (imagination)—create the base of a unified EF system. None can be logically understood as to how or why they exist without reference to the other two. Sensing the future cannot arise without self-awareness and self-inhibition, but the reason the latter two functions exist is to facilitate the third; alone these two would have no functional significance. Why be aware of and even stop yourself from doing something if there is no other course of action to be contemplated? The remaining EF components arise out of this triadic foundation—the development of speech and its eventual self-direction, the self-regulation of emotion and motivation, and reconstitution or play to the self.

It cannot be overemphasized that it is this capacity to contemplate one's goals and actions (ends and their means) across time that underlies much of the outward expansion of the extended EF phenotype into daily human life, community, and society. Other EF components clearly assist or abet that extension, but this is the primary driver of that extension. That is because it gives rise to the context of "later" that can be contrasted with the "now" and of a possible future against the current state. Most of the major domains of life activities in which humans engage, such as health maintenance, marriage, child-rearing, education, economics, ethics, law, and government, all depend as their starting point on this mental faculty—the capacity to contemplate, evaluate, and so appreciate the future consequences of one's actions *before* engaging in them. It provides the very reason to reciprocate, to cooperate, and to engage in mutualism (looking out for the interests of others besides your own) in daily human affairs. Absent this capacity to take "the long view" or consider the longer-term over which one is going to live, the individual degrades back to the automatic, impulsive, selfish, and often irrational level of behavior. If one cannot contemplate a possible future state, then there is no "later" to contrast with "the now" and hence no choice to be made and no need to choose—only to act so as to satisfy an immediate urge or relieve immediate uneasiness by the quickest means possible. Without a capacity for foresight, the future has no spokesperson or influence and cannot be maximized. An entity without a sense of the future is essentially blind to time.

Self-Directed Private Speech

Self-directed private speech is the alternative explanation for what cognitive neuropsychologists have called the verbal working memory system, particularly the phonological loop (Baddeley, 1986; Baddeley & Hitch, 1994). It is based on Vygotsky's theory of the internalization of speech (see Diaz & Berk, 1992) which forms the mind's voice used in verbal thinking. Individuals talk to themselves, often privately (mentally), to permit not just a private rehearsal of utterances (verbal simulations), though that is very important in its own right. The individual is using the same speech areas of the brain for this activity as they use when speaking publicly, except that the primary motor areas related to external or public speech are being suppressed (Ryding, Bradvik, & Ingvar, 1996).

As discussed in Chapter 2, language as communication or signal can be used to manipulate the behavior of another organism for the sender's own self-interests. When speech is turned back on the self, the signaler and the recipient are the same organism. Why would an organism seek to manipulate itself? It might need to do so if it had within its own skin (brain) a sense of two selves—the present self and the possible future self. The EF components that provide just such a bicameral self, as noted above, are self-awareness and self-directed sensing (hindsight and foresight). Self-speech also helps long-term self-interests to outweigh and replace short-term self-interests. The sense of the possible future gives rise to a sense of a future self, and it is that sense of the future that signals the present self to compete against its short term self-interests. Self-speech can be used as well to self-instruct and to self-question, and it can also be used for self-regulation, self-organization, and problem solving.

A capacity for symbolization and language is not an executive function, as defined here. It is associative. It is not a self-directed action, although the sensory–representational (visual imagery) system that gives rise to the icon to which the symbol refers is executive in nature because it *is* self-directed. Once a mental representation of a material thing can be prolonged, the image so held is capable of inducing the label or utterance for it. The person can now speak about things absent in the external world because they are using visual or other sensory imagery to drive the labeling (Deacon, 1997; Rossano, 2010). Then once language arose it gave humans yet another action that could be directed back on themselves—their own vocalizations. Symbolic language probably could not have evolved without first there being a means to mentally represent reality via self-directed sensory–motor actions (images) to which such symbols can now refer.

Labeling via language permits not only classification of things in the world, but a means for separating the various features of an object, such as size, color, density, temperature, spatial configuration, and movement. Once an object or action can be broken down in this way using language, more abstract concepts can be created out of these parts, categories, and classifications. Just as important, these parts can now be reconstituted to form entirely new entities that do not yet have any existence in reality; they are fabrications of the human mind using symbols (see Self-Directed Play below).

Self-Directed Appraisal (Emotion–Motivation)

Emotion is welded to everything we think, say, and do (Damasio, 1994). If individuals can redirect their sensing, saying, and doing back on themselves using the first four EF components above, this almost automatically grants them the capacity to elicit their own emotions and motivations. Emotions are short-term changes in our appraisal of events and are reflected in alterations in physiological arousal, perceptions of reinforcement–punishment (motivation), and hence, approach–avoidance behavior (Hess & Thibault, 2009; Neese & Ellsworth, 2009).

Because emotions are motivational states, they are also associated with the extent to which individuals increase or decrease their actions toward goals (Carver & Scheier, 2011).

This EF component is believed to initially arise as a consequence of the four above functions in which the individual comes to use self-awareness, inhibition, private imagery (and sensing more generally), and private speech to engender associated emotional and motivational states. The capacity to experience emotional states associated with information being held in mind, known as somatic markers (Damasio, 1994), provides a rapid means for calculating the costs and benefits to the individual of the imagined course of action and its goal. The means to goals are biologically costly in human effort and energy. They cannot be engaged in wantonly without some means of assessing the goal's value to the individual and the costs of the means relative to those goals. This EF component provides just such a cost/benefit calculator (self-appraiser) for mentally represented goals and the means needed to attain them.

Once humans developed a capacity to inhibit prepotent reactions to events and a capacity to contemplate "the later" against "the now," they automatically encountered a choice. As noted earlier, such a choice is inherently a conflict. A future state is being contrasted against the current one, and a decision must be made as to which is to be pursued. All such comparisons involve a calculation of costs and benefits for the individual. The goals (changes in uneasiness) to be gained from the possible choices are computed (valued) and then compared. The one producing a net maximization of value for the individual is then pursued. The decision is personal, reflecting the individual's appraisal of the subjective use-value of the means and ends. Therefore, a mental mechanism for the conscious executive appraisal involved in these comparisons must exist. It is argued here to be a component of EF. It provides for a rapid cost/benefit analysis of means and ends, and it appears to arise from bidirectional networks linking the dorsolateral frontal cortex, orbital-frontal cortex, anterior cingulated cortex, and amygdala (and hence limbic system)(Damasio, 1994, 1995; Etkin, Egner, Peraza, Kandel, & Hirsch, 2006; Ochsner & Gross, 2005, 2008; Ochsner et al., 2009; Rushworth, Behrens, Rudebeck, & Walton, 2007).

Injury to or disorders of the PFC (EF system) would therefore be expected to disrupt or distort this capacity for using mentally represented information for rapid appraisal of goals and means and hence how to value them. The problem can arise indirectly through injury to the system responsible for the creation of imaginary constructions (nonverbal and verbal working memory) or directly through the distortion, disruption, or disconnection of these systems from the emotional brain (amygdala and limbic system) via the anterior cingulate cortex. Damasio (1994) has eloquently described patients having disorders that disconnect or disrupt the system for mental representations from their emotional/motivational valences. The result is a significant inability to make decisions and choices about goals and means and to motivate the initiation of goal-directed actions.

The first four EF components can also be used for emotional self-regulation, the two-step process of initially inhibiting strong emotions and then downregulating or otherwise moderating them (Ochsner & Gross, 2005, 2008; Ochsner et al., 2009). Various disorders of the PFC result in an inability to self-regulate strong emotions that are not in the longer-term self-interests of the individual to display. Raw emotional displays, unmodified as to their appropriateness to a given social context, and poorly moderated are likely to impair social relationships, if not lead to outright rejection by others. Humans possess the means by which they can inhibit the initial displays of strong emotions. They employ these other EF components to replace the initial strong emotion with alternate emotional responses more consistent with social demands and the individual's goals and longer-term welfare. For humans, emotions are not merely environmentally provoked reactions that must be dealt with appropriately; they are also states that can be created *de novo* as needed in the service of one's goals (Izard, Stark, Trentacosta, & Schultz, 2008). This self-regulation of emotion is believed to be achieved by the same bidirectional network of connections that underlie the appraisal system for mentally contemplated goals and their means.

Because emotions are motivational states, this EF of creating private emotion and motivation probably also provides for the capacity for self-motivation—the drive states needed to initiate and sustain action toward the future. Recent research in neuroimaging and in developing rating scales of EF suggest that the emotion regulation and motivation regulation aspects of this unit may be partially separable both neuroanatomically (Murray, 2007; Rushworth et al., 2007) and behaviorally (Barkley, 2011a). Even so, they are treated as a single unit here for both the simplicity of presentation and because of their substantial neurological and functional overlap.

No matter how great the plan or mental map constructed to attain a goal, no self-powered, acting entity is going anywhere without a source of fuel. This is the drive, the will, or the motivation needed to sustain self-directed actions toward a future goal. The foregoing "cold" cognitive EF processes may be metaphorically compared to a computer brain in a modern self-guided missile. But that missile will not leave the launch pad without fuel. Such fuel may initially arise in large part as a consequence of being aware of the conflict between current wants and future desires and the magnitude of the disparity. Motivation may therefore reflect the initial strength of such desires and the emotional valence associated with one's needs (wants) and goals (desires). But long chains of hierarchically nested goal-directed action sequences take time and energy. The motivation needed to sustain such long-chain action plans becomes more crucial the longer the delay to the goal and the longer and more complex the action plan to achieve it. It is unlikely that initial motivational states can sustain such long-term action. There is an obvious need for a means of midcourse refueling—a conscious means by which the individual continually reenergizes the motivation needed for long-term, goal-directed actions. This EF component provides that source of internal fuel—self-motivation.

Self-Directed Play (Reconstitution or Problem Solving)

This EF is an alternative to the planning, problem-solving, and innovative (generativity/fluency) components noted in other views of EF. This component is hypothesized to be founded on the development of object play and pretense (symbolic play) in childhood (Carruthers, 2002). It is experimental in that the person is testing out "what if" arrangements of events and responses to them. It is regarded as reconstitution because it is essentially a two-step activity (Bronowski, 1977). The first is analysis, or taking apart features of the environmental contingency (event-response) and one's own prior behavior toward it. This is followed by synthesis or the recombination of components of both the environment and those behavioral structures that may be associated with it into novel arrangements. These novel combinations can then be tested out against a criterion, such as a problem or goal, for their likely effectiveness in overcoming obstacles to goal attainment. While this process begins in childhood as observable manual play, it progresses like the other EF components to being turned on the self and internalized as a form of private mental play. This permits both the manipulation of mentally represented information about the environment and about prior behavioral structures so as to yield new combinations that can serve as options for problem solving toward goals. It is possible that self-directed play can be subdivided into both nonverbal (ideational) and verbal (symbolic) modules that provide for fluency and generativity in each of these forms of behavior. Nonverbal, verbal, and action fluencies are believed to arise from this EF.

This type of play may have originated in the social play common to human children and the young of other species (Boulton & Smith, 1992). That form of play is typically practice or rehearsal of competition, aggression, cooperation, and compromise that may be needed at a later stage of maturation or by adulthood. But that sort of play typically does not have the analytic-synthetic process of experimenting with rearrangements of the environment to satisfy one's curiosity as to how such rearrangements might work. Humans engage not just in social play but in play with objects and eventually their cold cognitive mental representations that is the basis for problem solving.

Problem solving is often needed to begin a process of planning goal-directed action. That is because goal-directed action most often arises when there is a conflict between a present state (what is) and a desired state (what is wanted). Such a conflict, by definition, is a problem. Hence problem solving may be invoked at the very start of creating goal directed action. The problem-solving capacity provides for mentally creating and testing options for their likely ability to achieve the goal. This is predominantly a process of action fluency (Piatt, Fields, Paolo, & Troster, 1999), not so much object-naming fluency. In short, the individual can conceive of a variety of ways of doing something, selecting that which most likely will attain the goal given their experience. Evidence suggests that the orbital-frontal cortex and anterior cingulate cortex play distinct, yet interacting, roles in this process of generating and testing out a variety of response options (Rushworth et al., 2007).

Using this EF, humans discover new ways to reorganize components of the natural environment and of their own behavioral sequences. They do so to bring about new, better, or more efficient means to attaining human ends or goals and even new goals that could not previously be imagined. As the source of human innovation, this EF is akin to that of genetic recombination in the creation of gametes (eggs and sperm) that results in novel combinations of existing information encoded in genetic material. As the source of ideational and symbolic mutations and combinations, then, this EF permits a form of intrapersonal evolution (adaptation to the environment). At any level of universal evolution, to evolve new adaptations, mutations and combinations of existing information must be constantly offered up to the environment; from these the better adapted inventions are selectively retained and transmitted to the next trial (generation)(Dawkins, 1987; Mark Ridley, 1996). Self-play or reconstitution provides new ways of reorganizing existing mental information that lead to new ways of reorganizing one's behavior and environment.

Summary

To summarize, the EF components arise as a consequence of individuals turning upon themselves certain Pre-Executive level functions. By self-directing them, a person creates a capacity for self-awareness, self-modification, and self-regulation over time (future-directed, goal-focused, cross-temporal actions). Yet it is not just self-directed action that emerges here, but also a developmental internalization of those self-directed actions. This creates a conscious mental simulator—a mind. Why it would be necessary to keep one's self-directed actions private from others is an interesting question. It may be answered at the next level of EF's extended phenotypic effects where imitation and vicarious learning arise and thereby permit others as competitors to essentially plagiarize one's behavioral actions and innovations. This within-species competition would create the selection pressure necessary for driving the evolution of the internalization of self-directed actions. These evolutionary changes to the brain permit human choice and the direction of actions toward the future. At this level of the extended phenotype of EF—its creation—we can modify the initial phenotype of other animals to that of modern humans as follows:

genes → proteins & enzymes →
brain structures/pre-executive functions → covert self-directed actions

A self-directing, purposive primate with a sense of the future has arisen.

The Importance of Time in EF/SR

How We Derive a Sense of the Future

Self-awareness is a means for monitoring and evaluating what is initially automatic behavior at the Pre-Executive level. Once such automatic behavior is detected as being inconsistent with attaining a longer-term goal, self-awareness leads the individual to evaluate the situation that has transpired for clues. This is hindsight. The individual is looking back, re-sensing and even reverbalizing past events and his or her responses to them in order to guide readjustments to behavior in the next encounter.

A new hypothetical plan is constructed and stored for enactment when the event is next detected. Hindsight thereby leads to foresight; such foresight is the individual's best guess of what to expect on the next encounter, even when to expect it, and then how to respond. Repeated experiences with the situation can lead to fine tuning of the response. It may thus appear to others as if the person acts with clairvoyance when it is really with the hard-won knowledge from hindsight. On encountering a novel situation the individual has no idea what the future may hold. Yet he or she can activate hindsight of previous similar experiences for ideas on how best to act in this situation. The individual then uses the outcome of that encounter to readjust his or her subsequent behavior. The self-directed actions occurring at this level are thus teleological; they are purposefully implemented as means aimed at conjectured future goals.

For instance, when children talk to themselves while performing academic work, such as math problems on paper, such self-talk does not seem to initially benefit the current performance with that problem. Instead it correlates with improvement in subsequent encounters with that or similar problems (Diaz & Berk, 1992). In short, foresight emerges only as a function of self-monitoring of ongoing and largely automatic activities that can then be mentally reexperienced for further analysis (hindsight) when mistakes have been detected. Out of this a plan for adjusting behavior in the next encounter is constructed. Foresight is the product of that analysis and the hypothetical action proposed for use when encountering similar situations again.

Three Important Time Factors

The factor of time is inherent in human contemplation, valuation, choice, and actions toward goals. Three temporal factors are involved in such human choices and actions. The first is the temporal window defined as how far into the future the person can contemplate a possible goal; this is one's personal time horizon. The future being contemplated concerns only a particular goal and a specific context. The second factor is the time that goal-directed actions take to attain the goal. This is called "working time" by economists. It can be distinguished from the third temporal factor, which is the time period over which the attained goal is likely to satisfy one's uneasiness, known as the duration of serviceableness (Mises, 1990). All three temporal factors are important in human EF—in human contemplation, choice, and action.

Time, therefore, is essential to every act of reasoning that precedes and directs actions toward goals. A goal that takes a considerable working time and yet provides only momentary satisfaction of human wants is usually not worth pursuing. Likewise, a goal that takes little working time, yet results in a lengthy period of satisfaction, is usually highly valued and is often pursued. Individuals also vary in their preference for sooner versus later goals—that is, in their valuation of working time and of the duration of serviceableness. Overall, goals that can be obtained in less time than others are typically preferred. This is the concept of time preference in economics.

> The value of time, i.e., time preference or the higher valuation of want-satisfaction in nearer periods of the future as against that in remoter periods, is an essential element in human action. It determines every choice and every action. There is no man for whom the difference between sooner and later does not count. The time element is instrumental in the formation of all prices of all commodities and services. (Mises, 1990, p. 490)

There is considerable variation across people in their time preference, which is to say in their preference for nearer versus later consequences or inversely in their capacity to delay gratification. Future goals and consequences are steeply discounted as a function of their delay, all other factors being equal, and people vary in this degree of temporal discounting (Green et al., 1994, 1996; Mischel, 1983; Mischel & Ayduk, 2011). All of this is to say that an essential component in EF is that of time. It plays an important role in the contemplation of the future and especially in the appraisal or valuation assigned to means (working time) and ends (duration of serviceableness) and more generally to the total time between the decision to act and the attainment of the goal toward which it aims.

EF/SR Relies on a Limited Resource Pool

Researchers have long proposed that EF/SR is based on a limited resource pool of effort or willpower that can be depleted, replenished, or reduced or even boosted in capacity by various factors (e.g., protracted use of SR, exposure to reward or to visually imagined delayed rewards, brain injury, physical exercise, respectively) (Bauer & Baumeister, 2011). The pool is not only depleted by sustained engagement in SR in a given context, but by the use of any and all of the components of EF. This is to say that the pool is shared and nonspecific across various EF processes. It can also be depleted by illness and alcohol and drug use (Bauer & Baumeister, 2011). This pool appears to have some relationship to variations in blood (and hence brain) glucose levels (Gailliot & Baumeister, 2007) and can be replenished by consuming substances that contain glucose or boost blood glucose. The pool can also be refilled by engaging in various activities such as taking 10-minute relaxation or 3-minute meditation breaks, receiving positive rewards, and engaging in positive self-statements of efficacy after or even during sustained use of SR. And the pool capacity may even be boosted by the routine practice of EF/SR activities on a daily basis or by increasing routine physical exercise (Bauer & Baumeister, 2011).

Are All Self-Directed Actions EF?

It is important to appreciate that the private self-directed actions used for goal-directed behavior (EF) are considered to be executive *only* when all three of the components for defining self-regulation (SR) discussed above are met. Merely self-directing an action by itself is not EF/SR. Manually scratching an itch or singing to one's self privately (internally) in and of themselves would not be considered executive in nature, yet both are self-directed human actions. The self-directed action must also modify the subsequent human behavior from what it is likely to have been otherwise—it must be self-modifying. Yet meeting this criterion does not qualify a self-directed action as EF if the purpose of self-modification was not to be goal directed and focused on altering a future outcome for the benefit of one's welfare or satisfaction. For instance, I may daydream (self-directed imagery) while I should be working on a boring activity. My daydreaming alters my subsequent behavior from what it would have been otherwise. I am now less likely to get my work done in a timely fashion. But this is not EF because it is not directed intentionally at a goal or to alter a delayed consequence for my longer-term self-interests. Indeed, it has diminished my longer term welfare.

Self-directed private actions, such as self-speech and imagery, may well have evolved to allow and assist with action toward delayed goals and consequences, but once having arisen they can be used as ends in themselves (e.g., singing or talking to one's self for the sheer delight of doing so). That is not EF as it is not modifying subsequent behavior, and it is not goal-directed. Indeed, it may interfere with one's longer term goals and welfare. This may be the case with more pathological forms of mind wandering/daydreaming, as might be seen in ruminative disorders such as obsessive–compulsive disorder, and generalized anxiety disorder, or in the attentional disturbance known as sluggish cognitive tempo

(Barkley, 2012a). The fact that an action is self-directed and even mental in form does not make it useful for attaining one's goals and longer-term welfare; it is not an EF, and it may even be a perversion of EF, as in pathological mind-wandering.

This distinction is akin to the important distinction in economics between leisure and labor (Mises, 1990). Leisure is an end in itself, the pursuit of immediately pleasurable activities or at least activities that immediately reduce dissatisfaction. Labor is a means to a different and delayed end—a more mediate or delayed goal. Self-directed actions are EF when they are means to other ends. They are labor, not leisure.

This level of the EF phenotype makes clear what is contained in the traditional phrase of "the skills" or "processes" that support goal-directed behavior and problem solving used so often by others to define EF (see Chapter 1). Those neurocognitive processes are the private, mental, self-directed actions discussed above. They are called *self-directed* for the reason that it is the self-direction of pre-EF functions that defines an executive from a nonexecutive function or process. The nature of the constructs placed under the umbrella term of EF at this cognitive level, as described by others, also becomes clear. Each EF construct is a specific form of self-directed action (attention, imagery, speech, emotion, play, etc.). They are referred to as *processes* because they are not ends in themselves but means to higher order ends that are to be found at upper levels (and outer zones) of EF activity in daily human life. They are considered *instrumental* as they are necessary for generating the executive behavior that is used in daily life activities, but they are not sufficient for those higher EF levels to exist. In short, executive functions are conscious, volitional, purposive, effortful, self-directed teleological actions.

The neurocognitive instrumental–self-directed processes may possess a certain hierarchical structure within this level, as suggested in some earlier models of EF (Luria, 1966; Stuss & Benson, 1986) and in their developmental–sequential maturation as I previously theorized (Barkley, 1997b). But they are considered as a single level here because they are neither developmental nor evolutionary ends in themselves but serve higher levels of EF.

How Does EF Govern the Automatic Pre-Executive Level of Behavior?

SR (or EF here) has been usefully viewed by many different theorists as a two-level system (Carver & Scheier, 2011; Eisenberg et al., 2011;

Hofmann et al., 2011; Koole, van Dillen, & Sheppes, 2011; McRae, Ochsner, & Gross, 2011). The first level attends to "the now" and is automatic, pre-executive, unconscious, stimulus-driven, and largely reactive (Kahneman, 2011). It was discussed in the previous chapter. It is often focused on primitive features of the environment, both internal and external, and it is evident in other mammals. It involves a host of psychological abilities or evolved mental modules for situation detection, attentional control, event appraisal, and response generation. It serves to achieve immediate or near-term goals, and it largely focuses on the flow of events in "the now."

The second level is the executive, effortful, conscious one that attends to the future. It is the EF level that intervenes in and otherwise strives to regulate the automatic level in the service of longer-term goals across larger spans of time. It is focused on the flow of potential events lying ahead in the future, and it relies on mental representations (internal actions) to guide and adjust the motor system so as to alter the likelihood of potential future events. It seeks to wrest control of the "now" automatic system in the service of mental representations of longer-term goals and related information. This second level has a limited resource pool of strength or energy for engaging in acts of SR (Bauer & Baumeister, 2011), discussed above. It is within this second level that the EF components discussed earlier exist. They generate and sustain the mental representations that will cause the "top-down" regulation of the automatic level of human action (Badre, 2008; Banich, 2009; Botvinich, 2008; Hofmann et al., 2011). This top-down regulation can occur via at least five vectors of influence that are often used to describe how emotional self-control is exerted by the EF system. But they are just as useful in describing how all human action is guided by that system. These five vectors of influence are situation selection, situation modification, attentional redirection, event reappraisal, and response modification/suppression (Gross, 2007; Koole et al., 2011; McRae et al., 2011).

These five vectors of influence come from one of the most widely cited models of emotion regulation in the EF/SR literature—that of Gross (2007), known as *the modal model*. It specifies two types of action/emotion pathways (primary and secondary). There are four stages in the occurrence of primary actions/emotions: situation (event), attention, appraisal, and response. These were noted in the previous chapter as the pre-executive stages of information processing and action. The secondary or executive level action/emotion pathway may exert an influence over this primary pathway via five different vectors:

1. Situation selection: Choosing to enter or avoid situations that have been previously associated with strong primary emotions.

2. Situation modification: Electing to modify situations that previously have provoked strong emotions such that those emotions are less likely to happen, such as injecting artificial consequences into the situation to enhance emotional control, opting to place one's self in a different place in the situation near to others whose presence may facilitate SR, and so on.

3. Attention regulation: Using distraction or looking away, focusing attention away from the emotionally provocative stimulus, or focusing attention on certain "cold" informational features of the stimulus rather than certain "hot" or emotionally charged characteristics of the event.

4. Reappraisal: Rationally reevaluating the importance of the event, any detrimental effects an emotional response may have on goal-directed success, and other cognitive-behavioral techniques often used to reframe, reevaluate, or otherwise asymmetrically shift the importance of the event from the initial primary appraisal that evoked the emotion to the longer-term goals and welfare of the individual (Fishbach & Converse, 2011). This stage may even include employing thoughts, images, and private speech to generate a positive countermanding emotion that may serve to reduce or replace the initial primary emotion.

5. Response modification: The most effortful path of all. It usually consists of direct efforts to downregulate or even suppress the strong provoked emotions.

The first two vectors of SR described above are proactive in that they serve to head off the likelihood that the unwanted primary action/emotion will be experienced at all or make it more likely that a positive primary action/emotion will occur. The remaining three paths of top-down regulation are reactive in nature, occurring as they do after the primary action/emotion has been elicited. As McRae et al. (2011) describe this two-stage model of human emotion, efforts to self-regulate (intervene) earlier in the sequence, such as situation selection, are likely to prove more effective than are attempts at later stages such as response modification. The earlier paths for intervention are also likely to deplete the self-regulatory resource pool noted earlier less than are later ones (Bauer & Baumeister, 2011).

Although the model is often used to explain how people try to self-regulate strong negative emotional states, it also works well for explaining the SR of strong positive emotions. These can be enhanced and prolonged, if doing so is supportive of a goal, or downregulated if excessive for the specific context. One way to do so is by using cognitive devices such as mental contrasting—visual images of the desired state (goal) are simply contrasted with the current state. This alone has been shown to enhance or diminish motivation toward goals as well as the emotions associated with the current situation, thus making it a form of emotional self-control (Gollwitzer & Oettingen, 2011). Most likely this occurs because humans transfer the value of the goal to the means needed to attain it (Mises, 1990).

As others have noted (Fishbach & Converse, 2011; Mischel & Ayduk, 2011), SR (and so EF) is most often initiated whenever immediate desires conflict with more important longer-term goals. Resolving the conflict in favor of the longer-term goal demands SR (and so EF). Successful SR involves (1) identifying that a conflict between "the now" and "the future" actually exists and (2) asymmetric shifting of motivational strengths to favor the longer-term goal (and so diminish the natural tendency to discount the delayed outcome). Identifying that a conflict exists also involves (1) identifying and calculating the costs of each alternative for both the short term and long term; and (2) placing the immediate temptation in the perspective of a larger time frame (called width). Viewed in isolation, immediate desire poses no conflict. But it does when viewed as one event within a wider perspective on time, relative to other desires and over repeated instances. The wider the reference frame, the greater the likelihood of detecting such conflicts and so of initiating SR to combat them successfully. Asymmetric shifting of motivational strength from the immediate temptation to the longer-term goal, and so overcoming the automatic discounting of delayed consequences, requires a capacity for precisely those five vectors in the Gross model discussed earlier as pathways through which the executive control of emotion occurs. Once again, these are methods of situation selection, situation modification, attentional redirection, cognitive reappraisal (manipulating mental representations), and response modification/suppression. Failures in SR can arise not only from difficulties with shifting motivational strength. They can also arise from a simple failure to identify that a conflict even exists (Fishbach & Converse, 2011). And as noted above, once the future goal is deemed to be more valuable, the motivational shift toward the longer-term goal itself results in a transfer of that value or worth to the totality of the various means needed to achieve it.

Interestingly, the neural networks involved in efforts to self-regulate strong negative emotion overlap to some degree but not entirely with the neural networks involved in the upregulation of position emotion (McRae et al., 2011). But all of these neural networks overlap with or are identical to those noted previously as involved in EF (PFC regions, anterior cingulate cortex, basal ganglia, amygdala, cerebellum, and anterior corpus callosum). Using verbal reasoning and other verbal strategies as part of reappraisal activates the left lateral PFC typically associated with verbal working memory (or self-speech), while using distraction (attention regulation) activates a more limited region of the dorsolateral PFC as well as posterior attention orienting networks in the inferior parietal area. Distraction also appears to reduce amygdala activation better than reappraisal and even more so than response suppression, which has been shown to activate the amygdala further. Response suppression also appears to be mediated by the right lateral PFC, which is typically associated with inhibition of prepotent responses as well as the use of visual imagery specifically and nonverbal working memory more generally. In summary, there appear to be at least five vectors through which the EF system affects the automatic level of behavior through its use of the six self-directed EF components described in the model here.

Viewing EF/SR as a System of Feedback Loops

I have described EF as a set of self-directed actions that serve to initiate and sustain human action toward goals. Such a view is not incompatible with another model of self-regulation, known as feedback loop theory. This proposes that SR may involve a series of hierarchically organized feedback loops or control systems that serve to regulate goal-directed behavior just as they regulate motor actions (Carver & Scheier, 2011). The model argues that individuals hold in mind a goal and repeatedly compare their current status and actions against this goal to measure progress toward the goal and the rate of their progress. The disparity between current status and goal may be monitored by one mental system, while the speed of progress may be monitored by a separate system. The feedback from both systems causes course corrections and alters the velocity of progress. Emotional states are associated with variation in rates of progress toward goals. Slower than expected progress leads to emotions of frustration, anger, or hostility that motivate the individual to speed up progress, while evidence that the goal cannot be obtained may result in demoralization or depression and abandonment of the goal altogether. Progress that is faster than expected may lead to positive emotions. It may also result in a slowing or behavioral "coasting" toward the goal, given that effort can be reduced while still attaining the goal at the expected time. Feedback about the success of altering the rate of progress may then reduce the associated emotions. Such a model readily accounts for the striking variability in performance often associated with frontal lobe disorders, such as ADHD (Andreou et al., 2007; Gilden & Hancock, 2007). The model acknowledges that humans pursue multiple goals occurring at various levels of abstraction. Given this, a system is required that monitors the priority of the current goal and its actions and reprioritizes the various goals as needed, given new information obtained from the environment.

Carver and Scheier (2011) argue that emotions may not only serve to alter the pace of progress toward goals given feedback about it but may also initiate the reprioritization of goals. Negative affect signals a need to reprioritize current goals while positive affect may signal that a goal can be reprioritized downward or even abandoned if it has just been obtained. Complicating the model a bit further is the assertion that such a feedback loop system works at two levels. One is automatic, experiential, often unconscious, impulsive, and intuitive. It accounts for much routine behavior toward goals, especially those in the near term or those that recur and hence have relatively automatic behavioral programs. The second is effortful, conscious, deliberative, and rational. It is the executive level of goal-directed action that can alter or override the automatic level if one's actions have become inappropriate to the situation or consciously held goal. This second executive level consciously formulates abstract goals, which are usually longer term than those pursued at the automatic level. It also formulates the abstract principles needed to obtain those goals or subgoals. It then transfers this information to the automatic level for the execution of the more molecular sequence of smaller units of the plan. Actions aimed at emotional self-regulation also may be initiated from the executive level to deal with emotions that may be arising from the automatic level. Such a feedback control system view of SR can be readily mapped onto the components of EF as the need for inhibition, self-monitoring, working memory, planning/problem solving, and emotion regulation processes is readily apparent in this feedback loop model.

Evolutionary and Developmental Considerations

The six EF components hypothesized to exist at this level of the extended phenotype of EF do not develop simultaneously. Some components require the existence of others to emerge and function. This probably reflects their sequence in the evolution of modern humans. Logically, self-awareness (self-directed attention) must predate or co-develop with inhibition (self-restraint) and sensory imagery (sensing to the self). Self-awareness alone, without the power to alter what the self is doing, seems a useless function. Inhibition, as noted above, is essential to stop processes occurring at the automatic, Pre-Executive level of behavior (situation–attention–appraisal–response). Self-directed actions cannot occur as long as actions are being automatically and continuously directed at moment-to-moment events in the external world. Inhibition decouples the event from the response to it, buying the time needed for executive self-directed actions. There seems little need to interrupt the automatic sequence if some alternative course of action is not going to be contemplated via ideational representations. It therefore seems a reasonable hypothesis that the first three of the EF components coevolved close together and so co-develop in the early developmental period of each child. These ideational sensory–motor structures are likely the basis for gestural communication, the first communication system in human evolution and development. The public repetition of self-directed behavior, or mimesis, is not just a means for the rehearsal of human actions (Donald, 1991, 1993); it is a form of communication because witnesses are capable of copying what they see. Kelly and colleagues (2002) have also argued that the development of nonverbal actions (sensory–motor) served as the first system of communication in humans and as a stepping stone to symbolic language.

Deacon (1997) has explained how this may have happened. The emergence of visual imagery in the species served as a requisite stepping stone for the emergence of language as a symbolic system. This is because words are arbitrary utterances that must represent something else for their meaning. Images and other mentally represented sensory impressions provide that semantic content. This sequence from gestural to symbolic communication is evident today in the development of language in human children; nonverbal gestural communication precedes and then is used in conjunction with words. The privatization of self-directed sensing and eventually of self-directed sensory–motor action would have provided a means for self-guidance using nonverbal rule-governed behavior and private rehearsal. It is comparable to but a predecessor of the functions of self-speech in self-regulation. All of this is to say that the emergence of the self-directed sensory—motor system (nonverbal working memory) likely predates that of self-speech (verbal working memory) in evolution and in development. There can be no doubt, however, that the eventual emergence of language and subsequently its self-direction to become private self-speech provided an additional, more efficient, and more fine-grained and precise means of self-regulation, goal discernment and directedness, and problem solving. It would have permitted self-description, self-instruction, self-questioning, and the other means of self-guidance as Vygotsky (1962) reasoned. Self-directed imagery and speech likely predate the emergence of the planning and problem-solving module of EF. The latter module manipulates the contents of the former, playing with them. Furthermore, symbolic thought can provide a means to more quickly test out information for its conformity to reality and selectively retain the successful trials. However, it is unlikely that this is the level of the EF extended phenotype that served as the basis for the evolution of EF. Many other species survive without an EF system. Natural selection likely does not operate at this instrumental—self-directed level of EF until this level impacts daily human actions, social functioning, mating, and self and offspring survival (Barkley, 2001).

Shifting Sources of Control of Human Behavior

With the onset of EF in child development, one should be able to witness a shift in the sources that direct human actions. These shifts are hypothesized here to occur along five continua and are likely to take the three decades needed for the executive system of modern humans to reach full neurological maturation. These shifts in sources of influence over behavior are:

- From external to internal (mentally represented) events
- From the temporal now to the hypothetical future
- From immediate gratification to an increasing valuation of larger delayed consequences
- From control by others to self-regulation
- From a noncultural to a cultural existence

The mature adult engages in acts of self-regulation to pursue future goals using mentally represented information to conceptualize and anticipate hypothetical futures. This is done to make choices between a current state and a future desired state. The imagined goal and its means give rise to purposive action and serve to sustain it across large spans of time. All this is done for the attainment of longer delayed consequences (goals) over smaller immediate ones. Given the reciprocal interplay of individual EF with culture, individuals also avail themselves of prior inventions (means) to attain their goals, contemplate new ones, and otherwise see to their long-term welfare. From this perspective, disorders of or injuries to the PFC retard or regress the progression along these continua and hence produce the serious and recognizable deficits in EF discussed in Chapter 1.

Conclusions

At this Instrumental–Self-Directed level of the EF phenotype, EF itself arises. EF here is argued to be a set of six self-directed, largely covert activities that arose from turning some of the pre-executive brain functions back on the self to create self-regulation. This allowed the individual's subsequent behavior to be altered and increases the likelihood of attaining a future goal. EF is self-regulation. It can now be defined as *the use of self-directed actions (self-regulation) so as to choose goals and to select, enact, and sustain actions across time toward those goals.* Humans employ at least six types of self-directed activities, which I believe represent the executive functions: attention, inhibition, covert sensory–motor action, speech, emotion–motivation, and play. A diagram illustrating this level of the extended EF phenotype appears in Figure 4.1. It portrays the model as a series of concentric rings or zones (left side) and a stacked hierarchy of levels (right side). The lower level of the hierarchy (Pre-Executive) precedes the higher level (Instrumental–Self-Directed), but they overlap in their development rather than being purely sequential in form. This is indicated by their stepped arrangement. Using the eight emerging EF developmental capacities discussed in Chapter 3, the present level can be characterized as follows:

• *Spatial.* The capacity to contemplate spatial distances over which actions can be directed to achieve geographically distant goals is now possible.

• *Temporal.* The use of hindsight/foresight and the contemplation

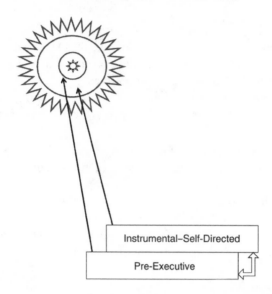

FIGURE 4.1. Two different ways of illustrating the extended EF phenotype as it occurs at the Instrumental–Self-Directed level. The concentric rings at the left indicate the outwardly radiating nature of the extended phenotype at this stage of development (Pre-Executive, Instrumental–Self-Directed). The starburst at the inner core of these rings represents the conventional view of a phenotype: genes → proteins → enzymes → structures/functions. The stacked boxes at the lower right label the levels and also indicate the hierarchical arrangement of two extended phenotypic levels beyond the conventional view. Information from the lower, Pre-Executive level flows upward to the higher, Instrumental–Self-Directed level, while that higher level may exert downward control to manage the lower level.

of a hypothetical future more generally bring into existence a conscious time horizon or temporal fore-period regarding the future (goals). In its initial development this may involve mere minutes ahead in time, but it eventually progresses outward from there to a few hours, a waking day, several days, and so on.

• *Inhibitory.* The ability to engage in executive inhibition or conscious self-restraint has arisen so as to decouple events from potential responses, interrupt the automatic flow of stimulus–response behaving, and provide for an opportunity to choose potential courses of action.

• *Motivational.* As a consequence of the former capacities, the value assigned to a delayed consequence has been increased (its reward value is not as steeply discounted as before). This leads to a motivational shift in the individual's preference of delayed rewards over immediate ones (from a higher to a lower time preference in economic terms). The individual is now increasing the subjective use-value of a delayed goal and is therefore more motivated by the prospect (mental contemplation) of such a goal.

• *Conceptual/abstract.* The capacity to self-direct speech and language provides the individual a means of using symbolic representations as a form of rule-governed behavior opening them up to all of the advantages that self-speech provides as noted above. Though such rules are necessarily simple, specific, and concrete in early development, with maturation there arises a capacity to guide behavior by longer, more complex, and more abstract rules. This gives rise to the conceptual/abstract capacity of the EF system.

• *Behavioral–structural.* The level of behavioral complexity needed here has increased by the added stage of the self-direction of actions. Behavior is no longer simple, automatic, and short-lived; it is now delayed, more complex, and deliberate. Alternative courses of action are being contemplated and are considered over a longer duration, giving rise to a need for a greater complexity of behavior so as to serve as the means to the goal and to bridge the delay in time to get it. Yet relative to higher level zones of the EF phenotype to be discussed next, such complexity probably still remains quite simple or low in degree, particularly in early child development.

• *Social.* The social complexity factor at this level remains very low in that there is little or no ongoing need for the individual to consciously plan to interact with and eventually use other members of the social group to operate at this level of EF. At this initial zone of the EF phenotype, the focus of action is self-directed.

• *Cultural.* The level of reciprocal influence with the culture is low, though not nonexistent. The flow of culture is largely one-way as EF develops—from social environment to child. Yet that inward flow of culture in childhood is massively assisted not only by parental instruction but also by participation in formal educational systems of pedagogy. The culture provides information and artifacts in the environment surrounding the individual that likely have some influence on the stimulation and growth, configuration, content, and purposes for which these initial executive functions are used. Compared to prior generations, culture can provide external scaffolding to ratchet up the individual's capacity for self-regulation over time toward goals. At the very least, culture can affect the content of one's mental representations (both visual–sensory and linguistic symbolic).

The next chapter extends the human EF phenotype to its next level and into everyday human life activities.

5

The Methodical–
Self-Reliant Level

The Instrumental–Self-Directed EF components described in Chapter 4 are largely covert, or private. This next level is concerned with human behavior; that is, observable everyday goal-directed actions. They are sustained, monitored, revised, and reprioritized by the lower or cognitive level of EF. At the Methodical–Self-Reliant level, the individual uses EF for daily survival that largely plays out in social settings. This level can be appreciated without having an exact specification of the components of the prior level. It is sufficient to assert that such an earlier "cognitive" level exists, is self-evident, and consists of various self-directed private activities used to mentally choose, simulate, enact, and sustain goal-directed actions. Extending the EF phenotype, the chain of effects now might look like this:

CNS pre-executive functions → CNS executive (self-regulatory) functions → executive (self-regulatory) adaptive behavior

The actions of other species, including other primates, are typically short-chained sequences for the attainment of rather near-term, quite proximal ends, often portrayed in stimulus–response contingencies and sequences. Actions are rarely if ever nested into sequences that involve subgoals, the attainment of which strung together can attain a larger, later-term goal. Humans, in contrast, engage in such nested sets of goal-directed actions as a matter of daily routine. A sequence of such actions or sets of actions strung together can be considered analogous to a recipe. No single action attains the goal but the set of actions completed in a particular sequence serves to do so. Here such a set of behavioral steps toward a goal will be called a method. A method is a procedure or process for achieving an end (Merriam-Webster, 1989) which accurately describes this "Methodical" level of the extended phenotype of EF.

This level is also titled "Self-Reliant" because it includes the daily routine activities (methods) that pertain to self-care and independence from others. It can be thought of as comprising the sorts of activities measured by those dimensions of adaptive behavior interviews and rating scales that pertain to the degree of responsibility individuals assume for fulfilling their own immediate and near-term (often daily) needs and wants. This includes assuming responsibility for sleeping, clothing and dressing, bathing and general hygiene, food or nourishment, personal safety and self-defense from the elements, from other species, and from other humans, shelter, and other self-care routines considered to be a necessary component of general self-reliance, survival, and basic social independence.

The Methodical–Self-Reliant level can be thought of as the "Robinson Crusoe" level of EF. It is not only comparable to the social isolation phase of the Robinson Crusoe story, in which he has no choice but to be self-reliant. It is also comparable to the later phases of that story when other methodical–self-reliant people arrive at his island with whom he must interact, yet from whom he must protect himself. The Machiavellian aspect to the story is applicable to this level of the extended EF phenotype. The basic background of any social ecology is competitive and predatory, whether it is between members of different species or between those of the same species. Self-interest prevails in all species as an inherent feature of genetics itself (self-replication) (Dawkins, 1976) as well as of the organisms created by those genes (survival, reproduction, and personal welfare). This level of EF accepts and respects intraspecies competition and predation as the background of humans just as it exists for all other organisms. Competition needs little explaining or justification. It is axiomatic; what requires explaining is the possibility that later levels of reciprocity and cooperation may emerge out of such interpersonal competition and inherent short-term self-interest (Axelrod, 1997).

The difference between the previous level and this Methodical–Self-Reliant one is analogous to learning to drive a car. It is one thing to be able to operate a motor vehicle in an empty parking lot but it's another thing to drive on the open road. Operating in the parking lot is comparable to the Instrumental–Self-Directed level of EF. The student driver is learning how to drive the car but is not driving to attain any other goal than practice. Driving on the highway is quite different because the driver is not only pursuing a goal but is also in the midst of other drivers pursuing their own goals and self-interests and with rules governing those interactions. Conflicts with others arise at many points of intersection. The first order of business for this driver is to drive safely, defensively and reach his or her destination while not interfering with or being obstructed by other drivers. This is precisely the stage of EF I wish to represent here, one of self-reliance with self-defense in pursuit of one's own goals.

Yet there is a nefarious aspect to this level that cannot go unremarked: group living provides the opportunity for individuals to prey on others for their own one-sided (parasitic) benefit. This opportunity exists across all species that encounter other living organisms within their range. As noted earlier, it also exists within the members of the same species, including humans. This is the very reason why individuals develop a form of social self-defense at this stage of EF while they too are capable of social parasitism. Some research even suggests that the extent of background risk of predation may be one force that leads to the evolution or adoption of cooperative strategies (Krams et al., 2009).

Parents and other adults appear to use artificially arranged consequences and other social and cultural scaffolding to assist children to successfully negotiate this stage of development as quickly as possible. Humans also may well have evolved certain social emotions such as shame, guilt, conscience, and empathy to further facilitate a quicker transition to the next stage of the EF phenotype. It remains, however, a stage to which individuals with PFC injuries may regress and out of which certain children with serious developmental disorders of the PFC/EF system may never fully progress.

Distinguishing Executive Cognition from Executive Action

It is at this level that thought and choice (covert EF) become action (overt behavior toward a goal). It will be useful in discussing this level of the extended phenotype to think of EF more broadly as comprised of both a covert and an overt level. At the covert level described in the last chapter, there exist private, cognitive self-directed actions that are largely mental (private) in form. By adolescence or adulthood, they are largely unobservable to others. These can be called *executive cognitions*

(EC), represented for instance by visual imagery and self-speech to plan and initiate goal-directed behavior as described in the last chapter. The overt, observable actions initiated and sustained toward goals may be thought of as *executive actions* (EA). Some EA may involve self-organizing the physical and social environment as discussed below and so are just as self-regulating as are the covert forms of EF or EC. Telling yourself in your own mind using self-speech to set your alarm clock at night is EC. Actually setting the alarm clock is an EA. In other words, EF can be bifurcated into EC that involve covert forms of SR and into EA that involve overt forms of SR. The latter is praxeological—that is, concerned with human action. EA may arise from having been chosen, initiated, and sustained by the covert mental level of EC. Henceforth I refer to EF in this broad sense of including both executive cognition and executive actions (EF = EC + EA). Even this distinction may eventually break down as advances in neuroimaging permit the observation of self-directed cognitive functions involved in EC. As noted elsewhere (Barkley, 1997b), the outward observable vestiges of EA in EC have already been detected.

Using the Physical Environment to Boost EF

A distinguishing feature at this level is the increased reliance on self-organized external props and other rearrangements of the physical environment that facilitate and even magnify the neurocognitive capacity for self-regulation across time. The individual interacts with the environment to create new products and methods (artifacts) that can serve as a means toward ends (goals). Humans produce new products and new methods for doing things by interacting with, taking apart, and recombining the elements of their physical environment. This is the human capacity for productivity (Mises, 1990). And so the concept of an extended phenotype as applied to this level of EF could be broadened from that shown at the beginning of this chapter to the following:

CNS pre-executive functions → CNS executive (self-regulatory) functions →
executive (self-regulatory) adaptive behavior →
new environmental arrangements (methods and products/artifacts)

Important at this level is human reorganization of the physical environment to facilitate self-regulation and goal-directed actions. This is evident in the human use of self-directed notes, written lists, clocks, calendars and other planners, computers and electronic schedulers, book-keeping systems, money, and simple rearrangements of the immediate environment such as placing an alarm clock by the bed and setting it. All of these and countless other self-directed props facilitate better self-management to time, self-organization, self-motivation, and personal productivity and so they help one to attain goals. Their effectiveness is clearly determined by how individuals self-arrange these physical components within their own life-space so as to increase self-regulation toward their goals.

For instance, the capacity to talk to oneself (an EC at the Instrumental–Self-Directed level) can be used to help organize and guide behavior over short-term intervals. Yet this control function can be extended a bit further across time and spatial distances when the individual speaks out loud, which is a stronger form of self-regulation—an EA. But the controlling effect of self-speech can be extended even further across space and time by creating a more permanent form of self-directed speech using written notes or other external self-directed props (another EA). These external recordings can encode the rules and instructions the person wishes to use in guiding his or her actions toward the intended goal. For instance, the "do list" that I keep on my desk along with my week-at-a-glance calendar of appointments and deadlines is far more effective at guiding my work-related activities for the week and month than if I had to rely on verbal working memory or self-speech alone.

Reliance on and off-loading of mental storage and work to such external devices massively boosts the storage capacity and complexity of information while effectively guiding individuals' behavior toward their goals. Those goals can exist at much further distances across space and time than was the case using just the internal mental means of representing information (the EC). Goals can be achieved with less time and effort, in many cases freeing up time and effort for pursuing other goals. This means that more goals can be pursued and attained; that, by definition, results in an increase in one's standard of living and hence long-term welfare.

This rearrangement of the physical environment to facilitate EF/SR and goal attainment is not merely moving things around that already exist in the physical environment, though it is clearly that. It also includes taking apart and recombining components of the physical world as a means of discovering and producing new, useful rearrangements—it is human productivity. This playful yet generative activity of analysis and synthesis into recombination initially arose at the instrumental–self-directed level of EF via internalized play (planning/problem solving). When this EC is extended outward to acting on the physical environment (EA), it can result in novel rearrangements that create new products and processes that attain goals not previously attainable. It is through such human productivity that innovation in goal-directed action is manifest in the material world. The manipulation of the environment through human effort to yield useful combinations (products) that serve to more effectively attain one's goals is the definition of production or productivity in economics (Mises, 1990) and philosophy (Piekoff, 1993). Both efficiency and productivity markedly increase at this level as a consequence of applying EF to environmental reorganization, and consequently so does one's standard of living, quality of life, and longer-term welfare.

Hence, unique to this extended phenotype model of EF is its specification of a level of EF/SR that involves self-structuring and self-organizing the physical (and later social) environment as a means to produce something of value. The procedure being used becomes, in economic terms, a means of production while the end of this process is the product so obtained. But products cannot only be ends or goals in themselves; they can also become means to other ends, as when a tool is invented to accomplish a further goal. Stored and communicated, such products, devices, and even methods or processes that are means of production become part of the cultural external scaffolding that can amplify the initial cognitive EF/SR system.

Social Problems That Likely Contributed to the Evolution of the Self-Reliant EF Level

Why would humans engage in rearrangements of their physical environment to create more efficient means of attaining their goals? No other species does this, or at least not to the degree seen in humans. The answer, I believe, lies in the group-living social niche in which humans evolved. Practically from birth we are surrounded by other self-interested, self-directed, goal-pursuing individuals. Their presence sets up at least three types of social selection pressures that are likely to have existed over human evolutionary history (and human development). I believe that this self-reliant level of EF/SR likely arose to address them. These pressures are: intraspecies competition, social predation, and vicarious learning. We will see that the three are related to each other and may have formed a common selection pressure that favored development of self-reliance as social self-defense. As others have argued, there is a social origin to self-regulation (Diaz, Neal, & Amaya-Williams, 1990).

Intraspecies Competition

It is self-evident that our fellow humans are our closest competitors for mates and resources necessary for survival. Yet we live in groups with other self-interested beings as we compete with them. Human cognition must possess certain mental faculties that help to deal with this competition. Social life speeds up the rate of change in the environment. The early levels of universal evolution would simply not be rapid enough to permit adaptations to arise to it. Genetic evolution has been capable of adapting species to the physical environment over geologic time scales. As living entities found themselves dealing with other organisms in that environment, operant conditioning arose to permit a more rapid pace of behavioral adaptation. A new and even more rapid level of change arose in the social environment as earlier species of humans found themselves living with other humans who were self-directing, purposive, goal-oriented, and against whom they had to compete. One basis for the evolution of EF, I argue, is that it provided the means of more rapidly adapting to the flux, vexations, and uncertainty inherent in social conflicts.

Self-Defense from Social Influence, Persuasion, and Coercion (Social Predation)

Social existence guarantees competition for limited resources. Competition means that individuals will attempt to influence others for their own one-sided benefit and self-interests. It is social parasitism or predation. This occurs very frequently in the biological world within and between species, as discussed in Chapter 2. Human communication systems such as gesture and language serve just this purpose—to alter the mental representations and behavior of others for one's own ends or purposes. Not all efforts at social influence are parasitic or detrimental to the person targeted. For example, communication among genetically related individuals tends to promote inclusive fitness of the shared genotype (genetic self-interests) as would be expected from selfish gene theory (Dawkins, 1976). But we must accept the fact that in the biological world, many such communicative systems are parasitic or one-sided in promoting only the self-interests of the signaler to the detriment of the recipient. Thus some means of resisting, repelling, or just delaying and further evaluating such influences will be essential to the individual's welfare.

Mental mechanisms, such as self-regulation and other forms of resistance to unwanted, detrimental social influences are needed to counter this manipulative aspect of human social life. The efforts of people to influence others into giving up valuable resources are evident not only in advertising, marketing, and salesmanship, but also in such activities as theft, embezzlement, and financial scams. Advances in telecommunications such as the Internet have only broadened the opportunity to communicate, sell, persuade and swindle, and otherwise prey on others for one's own one-sided benefit.

An example of the Machiavellian side to the extended EF phenotype appeared in my local paper (Shiffer, 2011). A woman in Burnsville, Minnesota, was defrauded of $10,000 through an Internet dating website. The 53-year-old woman was matched through the website with a man misrepresenting himself as a businessman from Maryland. Over 3.5 months, their friendship blossomed into romance via e-mail, text messaging, and even telephone calls. Eventually, he asked her for a loan of $10,000 to address an emergency in his business situation. She provided it, only to discover shortly thereafter that the man was a Nigerian scammer. She lost all the money. Such scams are widespread, and they illustrate the long reach of the EF phenotype (and its genes). It is my contention that the Methodical–Self-Reliant zone of the EF phenotype arose in large part to address social parasitism enacted via persuasion, manipulation, and even coercion.

Remember from Chapter 2, that variations in genes and genotypes can exist in some organisms for behavior that serves to manipulate other organisms. Those other organisms then develop adaptations to defend against such manipulations. This can result in an arms race between phenotypes. Each genotype contains variations to deal with nefarious behavioral (and hence genetic) variations in the competitors. But variation will not just be at the genetic level (Dawkins, 1982). Variation at all levels of universal Darwinism can be expected to arise in response to human manipulations; as a consequence, there is variation in modes of thinking and in cultural rules. We are no exception to this circumstance.

Through the development of self-regulation, as discussed in Chapter 4, individuals progressively shift from being controlled by others to one's self as the source of control. This shift protects and enhances one's own self-interests. By becoming self-directed and self-reliant, the person is less subject to the manipulations, persuasions, coercive actions, and general social predation of others that would be detrimental to his or her short- and longer-term welfare. Therefore, with the emergence of the EF system, there should appear a growing resistance to social influence coupled with a growing capacity for self-determination. Eventually (as EFs mature through the three phenotypic levels that follow), the individual becomes free to choose with whom to reciprocate and cooperate in more symbiotic, mutually beneficial arrangements.

Imitation and Vicarious Learning

Living with others affords opportunities to observe and learn from their trial-and-error performances. This is vicarious learning and probably evolved from the visual imagery component of EF discussed in the last chapter. Such images of the behavior of others serve as templates for copying. From an evolutionary perspective, it would be incredibly beneficial to an individual's welfare if he or she had the capacity to copy the successful trials of others. But if individuals can copy each other's actions, then person A can alter what B is likely to do next simply by what A elects to do. This sets up a means for them to mutually influence each other's behavior. Such influence becomes a form of signaling or communication using behavior; it can become gestural communication.

Recall in Chapter 2 that methods of signaling or communication do not tend to arise for the benefit of groups but rather for the self-interest of individuals. More complex communication by gesture can arise because it permits one individual, A, to manipulate the mental representations and subsequent behavior of another, B, for A's own ends and not for the advantage of B. Certainly mutual benefit, too, can occur and likely facilitates communication among genetically similar individuals (kin) who have shared genetic self-interests. Regardless of its origin, this capacity of individuals to copy each other's behavior and then to influence each other by gesture means that there is genetic variation in each individual that explains behavioral variation in another person. Dawkins (1982) predicted this would be the case from his extended phenotype viewpoint. I am aware of no behavioral genetic research that has explored this likely possibility.

Eventually the capacity to imitate another could lead to the opposite—a capacity to act in opposition to what one sees by suppressing one's own behavior when observing mistakes in such trials. If you can influence what I do because I can copy your actions, that influence is not always in my best interests. It could be to my detriment if you are trying to manipulate my behavior for your own ends and welfare. Such imitation and the crude method of communication it affords might well set up a selection pressure to be more selective in what behavior is imitated or treated as a signal. Indeed, it may be in my own best interests to do the opposite of what you have done, especially if what you are doing is likely to be unsuccessful or risk personal harm.

However they arose in evolution, both imitation and vicarious learning are forms of experiential plagiarism that would save a great deal of time and energy relative to Skinnerian trial-and-error learning. Once visual imagery and related private sensory–motor action evolved, they could provide the mental template for copying observed actions and their consequences. Given intraspecies competition, this would likely lead rapidly to the development of an ever greater capacity to copy the learning experiences of others along with a pressure to keep one's own trial-and-error performances to one's self (Dugatkin, 2000). That privatization would preclude actions from being plagiarized by others, thereby avoiding losing one's competitive advantage over them. As I have previously argued, this may well have been the selection pressure that drove humans to evolve private, internalized system for behavioral simulation—the internalization of action so as to prevent experiential plagiarism by one's human competitors (Barkley, 1997b, 2001).

The neurological mechanism for this mental capacity is the mirror neuronal system of the prefrontal cortex (Rizzolatti & Craighero, 2004; Rizzolatti, DiPellegrino, Fadiga, Fogassi, & Gallese, 1996; see also van Leeuwan et al., 2009). Studies show that the capacity to imitate the actions of others is now virtually an instinct at the level of neuronal functioning. The PFC responds to viewing others' actions by activating the same sensory–motor regions of the brain as the acting person is using to create that behavior. This mirror–neuronal system has been linked to theory of mind and to empathy, among other human mental attributes related to EF. Yet modern neuropsychological cognitive models of EF or its psychometric assessment make no mention of imitation, vicarious learning, or even the possible development of theory of mind as being involved in EF. Nevertheless, vicarious learning is the starting point for culture—for the spread (replication) of information across individuals. While the capacities for language and verbal working memory serve to greatly expand the human capacity for adopting from and contributing back to culture, imitation is culture's starting point.

Note that the expansion of the EF system for these new purposes would likely lead to amending the existing six EF components described in the previous chapter to assist with *theory of mind* (which has been linked to EF via the processes of inhibition and working memory [Carlson, Moses, & Breton, 2002]), and *vicarious learning* subserved by the mirror–neuronal regions of the PFC and undoubtedly facilitated by the evolution of visual imagery or nonverbal working memory as noted above (Barkley, 1997b).

As discussed in the previous chapter, the combination of a capacity to rehearse one's behavioral performances for practice that can arise from the EF component of sensory representations to the self (nonverbal working memory) along with the capacity to imitate the actions of another such visual imagery provides can create a system of nonverbal signaling–gestural communication. Such a signaling system is a force for both good and evil. It can be used to signal genetically related individuals (family members) for the good of all (mutual symbiotic communication). But it can just as easily be used for parasitism, or the manipulation of unrelated others to one's own advantage for purposes of one's self-interests.

Dimensions of EF Evident in Daily Life Activities

It is at the Methodical–Self-Reliant level that rating scales of EF in daily life are likely to prove far superior at capturing the nature of the EA and their deficits than any EF test could possibly achieve. EF tests and EF rating scales are not in competition with each other; rather, they are different means of assessing *different levels* of EF in human affairs. Tests sample moment-to-moment instrumental (cognitive) EF processes (EC); ratings sample methodical EF behavior over hours to days and even over weeks at a time across multiple situations including social ones (EA). Therefore, the choice of which measurement method to use is dictated by the purpose of the evaluation and the level of the EF extended phenotype one wishes to assess.

What do such rating scales reveal as being the likely EA that exist at this Methodical–Self-Reliant level? Research on the Behavior Rating Inventory of Executive Functioning—Child Version (BRIEF; Gioia et al., 2000) shows an initial nine subscales of their scale. But these subscales were organized by the developers based only on the face validity of items and their similarities. When statistical methods are applied to these scores to identify their underlying dimensions, as in factor analysis, these subscales actually reduce to a two-dimensional structure. The first dimension is called metacognition and contains scales that assess working memory, time management, organization, planning and problem solving, and related abilities. The second dimension reflects behavioral regulation (inhibition) and comprises items that pertain to impulse control as well as emotional control and self-restraint. This factor structure also emerges in the subsequently published adult version of this scale (BRIEF-A; Roth et al., 2005).

My own research employed the initial version of the Deficits in Executive Functioning Scale (DEFS; Barkley, 2011a; Barkley & Murphy, 2010, 2011) with clinic-referred samples of adults with ADHD, adults with other disorders, and a general community sample. It revealed that the initial 91 EF items when subjected to factor analysis resulted in five factors. Noteworthy is that the first factor accounted for the majority of variance before rotation (more than 40%) and was labeled as Self-Management to Time. A similar factor was identified in research by two other teams using this same prototype EF scale (Biederman et al., 2007; Fedele, Hartung, Canu, & Wilkowski, 2010). It most likely corresponds to the metacognitive factor on the BRIEF. The second factor was Self-Organization and Problem Solving, which would also seem to be highly related to the Metacognitive dimension of the BRIEF-A. The remaining factors were Self-Restraint (inhibition), Self-Motivation, and Self-Activation and Concentration, all of which are likely related to the Behavioral Inhibition Dimension of the BRIEF-A. The factors on the DEFS were highly intercorrelated (.70 or greater), yet each contributed some unique variance to EF apart from their substantial shared variance. This substantial degree of shared variance was interpreted as reflecting an underlying metaconstruct of EF, similar to g in the field of intelligence (Barkley & Murphy, 2011). It most likely in this sample represented the EF of self-management across time as Fuster (1997) argued to be the overarching function of the PFC. Yet the smaller additional factors seemed important to identify as providing additional explained or unique variance in EF in daily life activities. As others (Miyake et al., 2000) have noted, even at the instrumental cognitive level EF appears to have unity-but-diversity.

Of course, the rating scale lacked items dealing with emotional self-regulation, and so no factor reflecting this EF would emerge in that analysis. Yet such a factor did emerge in the final version of the DEFS once such items were added (Barkley, 2011a). I subsequently collected normative information on the revised final version of the DEFS using a large representative sample of U.S. adults ($N = 1,240$). In that sample, the following five factors emerged, four of which were present in the earlier prototype scale: Self-Management to Time, Self-Organization and Problem Solving, Self-Discipline, Self-Motivation, and Self-Regulation of Emotions. But in this sample the factor of Self-Organization and Problem Solving accounted for the most variance before rotation. This contrasts with the earlier research on ADHD that found Self-Management to Time to be the largest factor. All this implies that in the general population, Self-Organization and Problem Solving accounts for the most variance in EF in daily life, but in ADHD, the greatest variation among adults with and without the disorder is one of time management. Research therefore suggests that at the Methodical–Self-Reliant level of EF, between two and five dimensions of EA can be identified. These are largely not being sampled by EF tests at the instrumental cognitive level or at least not very effectively.

EF as Human Reasoning and as the Source of Culture

EF at the Instrumental level can be usefully construed in layperson's terms as *reasoning*; it is the creative engine of culture. Reason deals with discerning the means for attaining ends (Mises, 1990, p. 173). The EF components are the mental faculties that are its basis; in lay terms, they are *thinking*. Using EF, individuals observe, conceptualize and propose, evaluate and criticize, discern, experiment, and otherwise problem-solve and invent new means of attaining their goals and seeing to their long-term welfare. They then engage in rearrangements of the physical environment to assist their goal-directed actions. Many of these new means to attain ends are in the form of recorded information, products, and other cultural artifacts that spread beyond the individual and even the immediate social group and may endure beyond the individual's own lifetime. These cultural products can then feed back to benefit the individual and feed forward to benefit others currently and in subsequent generations by providing cultural scaffolding for their own EF/SR and goal-directed actions.

Culture is a form of universal Darwinism, as discussed in Chapter 2. It is another mode of inheritance for humans and for their adaptive success beyond genetics and operant learning. Culture arises from individuals using EF (thinking and reasoning) to invent new devices, products, or other means of achieving ends and then transmitting them within and across generations. This precludes the need for every generation to start from scratch and reinvent old wheels. It is an exceptionally efficient and effective form of informational evolution because it can rapidly improve the adaptive and reproductive success and welfare of those creating it and those who are recipients of it. In short, the exchange between EF and culture is reciprocal or bidirectional. EF is needed to create culture, and EF uses the surrounding culture to ratchet up greater capacities for self-regulation toward goals, greater and longer-term goals, and a greater likelihood of achieving them.

Conclusions

With what has been learned above, we can now amend our definition of EF as follows: *the use of self-directed actions (self-regulation) so as to choose goals and to select, enact, and sustain actions across time toward those goals **usually in the context of others**.* One can illustrate this level of the extended EF phenotype as shown in Figure 5.1. Once more, this diagram reflects the phenotype as a series of concentric rings. A new ring has been added that corresponds to this newly emerged Methodical–Self-Reliant level. The right-hand side of this diagram labels the rings while also depicting them as a series of hierarchically organized levels that interact with each other.

The eight developmental capacities expand at this level as fol-

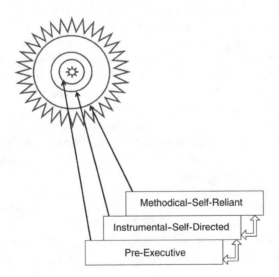

FIGURE 5.1. The concentric rings indicate the outwardly radiating nature of this Methodical–Self-Reliant stage of development (Pre-Executive, Instrumental–Self-Directed, Methodical–Self-Reliant). The stacked boxes at the lower right label the rings as well as indicate the hierarchical arrangement of the three phenotypic levels. Information from the lower level flows upward to the higher level, while the higher level may exert downward management of the lower levels.

lows. The *spatial* distances over which the individual contemplates goal-directed action increases. The invention of maps in the culture would have greatly boosted this initial capacity. The *time* horizon being employed to contemplate future events may be hours to a few days. The invention of timekeeping/recording devices in the culture would have greatly boosted this capacity. The extent to which the individual values future rewards (*motivation*) has increased accordingly, and reward discounting has decreased. The cultural invention of money and arithmetic would have greatly boosted this capacity to appraise the values of various goals and means, facilitating the cost/benefit analysis of each. The degree of self-restraint (*inhibition*) needed to achieve this level has also expanded from that required at the previous initial EF level. There is still a need to subordinate one's immediate selfish interests to one's delayed, longer-term future self-interests if one is to succeed at self-reliance. The degree of *abstract or conceptual* rules being followed has increased from the prior level as individuals invent and adopt spoken and written rules to guide their daily activities. The level of *behavioral* complexity operating here is greater than previous levels but is low in comparison to the next level described in Chapter 6. Certainly, more complex and nested sets of hierarchically organized action sequences are needed here than at lower levels as when making meal preparations for the day, shopping for groceries, making a bank deposit, planning out the course of a driving trip, and the like. *Social* interactions with others are simple ones that occur mainly in passing during daily encounters with others. But at this level the individual is not yet relying on those others to achieve near-term goals. This level of EF may have arisen as a source of social self-defense against the competitive and mutually manipulative features of the social environment, hence my emphasis at this level on self-reliance. Involvement of others is largely one of competition for resources or other valuables. Finally, the degree of *culture* being used here is greater than at prior levels but is likely to be only at the level of protoculture such as seen in earlier, primitive tribes of humans or even prehumans, perhaps such as Neanderthals. That culture consists chiefly in copying the behavior of others for self-benefit and in practicing a primitive form of gestural and possibly vocal communication. But it can also include the creation and adoption of relatively simple tools, weapons, and other useful artifacts.

6

The Tactical–Reciprocal Level

The Tactical–Reciprocal level described in this chapter represents the extension of the Instrumental–Self-Directed and Methodical–Self-Reliant levels of EF upward and outward into daily human *social* reciprocal or symbiotic relationships. At this level, the individual incorporates the use of others and social interactions with them as tools or means for the attainment of a goal. However, the use of others is no longer parasitic but symbiotic, of mutual benefit through social reciprocity. The evolution of cooperation among self-interested organisms has been a problem requiring explanation throughout much of the history of the theory of evolution. Thirty years ago, a solution was proposed that shows how such reciprocity can evolve among self-interested organisms, be beneficial to both, and remain stable over time even in the absence of an EF system (Axelrod, 1997; Axelrod & Hamilton, 1981). It is most likely to evolve in genetically related individuals as a starting point (known as kin selection), but it can occur among unrelated individuals if certain conditions exist (Michod, 1999; Nowak, 2006). I am here proposing that to develop in unrelated individuals, some psychological mechanism must exist to create and support this social activity, which I hypothesize is the EF system.

In the present model, this level of reciprocity comes into being in humans because of at least four factors:

1. The greater capacity of the individual to contemplate events, goals, or end-states at a greater distance across both space and time than was necessary for the functioning at the lower EF levels
2. The proximal availability of other self-directing, self-reliant individuals who can do the same (contemplate the longer term)

3. The attainment of a relative stalemate in the arms race that likely ensued at the next lower EF level from mutual predation or social parasitism (social parasitism becomes a less successful strategy)
4. The evolution of social emotions that promote reciprocal, symbiotic, and cooperative social behavior

The combination of these and probably other factors creates the opportunity for mutually beneficial reciprocity or social exchange to be discovered and utilized as a means that each individual in the exchange can use to his or her own self-advantage.

This new social realm of EF is an important one but is often overlooked in the contemporary literature on EF except by a few others such as Eslinger (1996) or Lezak (1995), and more recently Rossano (2011) in the cognitive control literature. However, it was well recognized in the literature earlier in the 19th and 20th centuries concerning the consequences of PFC injuries in humans (Harlow, 1848, 1868; Luria, 1966). It has also been duly noted in the literature on self-regulation (Finkel & Fitzsimons, 2011; Fitzsimons & Finkel, 2011; McCullough & Carter, 2011). And neuroimaging studies have shown that the use of reciprocity (McCabe, Houser, Ryan, Smith, & Trouard, 2001) and conditional cooperation in humans is mediated by the PFC (Suzuki, Niki, Fujisaki, & Akiyama, 2011), as well as other EF networks interacting with the PFC, such as the anterior cingulate, caudate nucleus, and nucleus acumbens (Rilling et al., 2002). Reciprocity (and the next level, cooperation) may involve a combination of theory of mind, cost-benefit calculations, and inhibition of the propensity to cooperate when faced with a noncooperator (McCabe et al., 2001; Suzuki et al., 2011). These social levels of the extended EF phenotype serve to emphasize the serious social deficits likely to occur from injury to or disorders of the PFC.

With maturation, the individual is capable of discerning goals across a longer term and at a greater spatial distance. This expanded temporal/spatial horizon results in a greater motivational valuation of events further out in space and time than was the case at lower levels. It also results in a capacity to contemplate a longer sequence of actions, including intermediate goals with their nested sets of actions that, when strung together, can attain the longer-term goal. This expanded capacity for forethought also permits the individual to contemplate the effects of one's behavior on others and of their behavior on him or her. There is a point in the temporal extension of foresight where one can appreciate the fact that the longer-term self-interests of individuals begin to converge. The invoking of verbal rules may further assist the bridging of actions across time and space, as might the creation of more abstract, conceptual rules. Each of these may represent subsets of more specific rules. The use of cultural products, discoveries, or inventions also becomes increasingly important as a means toward goals. As noted in previous chapters, this important impact of cultural scaffolding will increase at each movement upward and outward of the remaining levels of the EF extended phenotype.

This level is termed *tactical* because individuals will need to develop sets of methods—shorter-term behavioral means and goals—to achieve longer-term goals and higher order. That pursuit is being conducted in the midst of other self-regulating individuals. Self-defense and self-reliance were the first order of social business at the earlier level. Here, however, the individual contemplates the possibility that others can be used in a mutually beneficial way to facilitate one's own goals. At the earlier self-reliant level, individuals rearranged the physical environment to promote their own goal-directed activities; at this level, individuals are now going to organize the social environment to do so.

This level of EF is also termed *reciprocal* because the individual is now not just relating to others by chance in passing during daily activities. The person also is not just defending against the pernicious social influences of others as in social parasitism. At this level, an individual is *utilizing* others, with the others' consent, to pursue longer-term goals— goals that cannot be achieved as efficiently alone and that are mutually beneficial. This utilization of another person is not necessarily one-sided, parasitic, or short-term selfishness. It is more commonly symbiotic and reciprocal, involving mutual consent in the service of each person's *longer-term* self-interests. Each benefits from the interaction to a degree that they could not do so as effectively or efficiently alone. When each person understands and pursues his or her self-interests over a longer time frame, such self-interests can be seen to converge and be similar if not identical. Only an expansion in the developmental capacity to foresee consequences at a greater spatial and temporal distance *and across social others* would permit the individual to voluntarily and consciously recognize the larger value of reciprocity over individualistic and autarkic action alone. This is the basis of ethics (morality) (Hauser, 2006; Hazlitt, 1998) including *the Golden Rule*. At the previous level the individual sought to organize the physical environment for self-regulation and goal-attainment; at this level the individual is starting to organize others to achieve the same result. But the decision to reciprocate with others is always conditional, based on information about the setting and especially the other individual, the signals they may give as potential reciprocators or cheaters, and their reputation (Axelrod, 1997; Suzuki et al., 2011).

The extended EF phenotype at this level may be diagrammed as follows:

CNS pre-executive functions → CNS executive (self-regulatory) functions →
executive (self-regulatory) adaptive behavior → self-organization
of environmental arrangements (methods, products, artifacts) →
self-organizing of social arrangements to achieve
reciprocal exchanges with others

Social Reciprocity as a Major Activity of the Extended EF Phenotype

A hallmark of this level is engagement in social reciprocity, known also as reciprocal or social exchange. Why would it arise? It is because individuals have things (goods) or do things (services, etc.) that others may value. Given the natural variation in physical resources—hence the variation in their availability to individuals—and the natural variation in human abilities, some things may be produced in excess. Individuals therefore can exchange their excess items for others of comparable or greater value to mutual benefit as they perceive that benefit to be (subjective use value). Bartering and trade seen at this level is not just an essential beginning component of human economic activity; it is also a principal means of human survival.

Reciprocity goes beyond just trading products; it also forms a part of human social interaction. It involves social etiquette and skills in which individuals engage in small favors and courtesies with an expectation of reciprocity now or later, even if the response is only an expression of gratitude. Taking turns, sharing, and other such reciprocal social behaviors emerge in the late preschool and early elementary years of children, with strong training and encouragement by parents, teachers, and others in society. About the same time, there emerge theory of mind and the social emotions, probably because they are essential to the existence of reciprocity. Etiquette can be likened to a form of "social grease" that can make the myriad of social encounters and interactions run more efficiently and smoothly, with less conflict, than would otherwise be the case. And it can make those on the receiving end more likely to reciprocate. Driving rules, like social rules, often rely on reciprocity to reduce the probability of conflict. Turn-taking at intersections, for instance, allows all drivers to get to their destinations more quickly, with less conflict. The same applies in the larger domain of social interactions. Reciprocity in social interactions reduces conflict and permits participants to be more likely to get to their goals and do so more quickly while doing so in the context of other goal-pursuing self-regulating individuals.

Initially, the individual goals being pursued at this level may be relatively simple ones of short-term duration. A tactical EF suffices to achieve a near-term goal that may be just hours away. As this level develops, however, these tactics may be aimed at somewhat longer-term goals within the same day or the next few days. It all depends on how far out in space and time the individual is able to contemplate the future and the effects of any tactics. Also emerging is a capacity to look across *social distances* (across people) to contemplate possible reciprocal exchanges that may facilitate the achievement of one's goals.

From Rearranging the Physical Environment to Rearranging the Social One

A distinguishing feature of the previous Methodical–Self-Reliant level was the use of external physical props and other rearrangements of the environment that would facilitate self-regulation across time. As one moves upward and outward to the Tactical–Reciprocal level, these external means of self-management involve using others to further extend the spatial and temporal range of self-regulation and hence of goal attainment.

For instance, someone may wish to increase the frequency of their exercising for better health or weight loss. To better achieve that goal, they arrange to have a neighbor who is also a runner meet them each morning before work to run together. Both benefit from this exchange. This is not cooperation, which arises at the next level. It is reciprocal self-regulation in which each person seeks out the other to hold them socially accountable for a behavior-change program that they are far less likely to successfully engage in had they just tried to do it on their own (Finkel & Fitzsimons, 2011; Fitzsimons & Finkel, 2011; McCullough & Carter, 2011).

The individual may also arrange for others to assist with trading, improving work productivity and meeting goals for a promotion, improving or changing career paths, managing and saving money, health maintenance, weight loss, substance management and reduction (i.e.. quitting smoking), pursuing further educational degrees, participating in community activities, and so on. This is not a form of social dependence, which is a one-sided reliance on others to do things for you. It is instead a mutual reliance in the service of exchanging resources and other valued assets. It is symbiotic when it works well and it is parasitic when it does not. In short, the individual is not just rearranging the nearby spatial environment to facilitate self-regulation and goal attainment, as at the Self-Reliant level. Such individuals are now rearranging the *social* environment to further assist with both self-regulation and with goal pursuit and attainment.

The Special Conditions Needed to Support Reciprocity

This Tactical–Reciprocal level likely evolved to solve important adaptive problems caused by living in groups. These problems and related opportunities probably posed evolutionary selection pressures for which the Instrumental–Self-Directed and Methodical–Self-Reliant levels of EF do not seem completely suited. A third level of EF/SR would need to eventually emerge: the Tactical–Reciprocal one.

Acts of reciprocity are known to arise in highly genetically related individuals that reside in groups, as in ant colonies, without the need for any EF or even consciousness to support them. Selfish gene theory (Dawkins, 1976) and related concepts of kin selection (Krebs, 1998; Ridley, Mark, 2001) would lead to genes for unconscious altruistic behavior to emerge as a function of the degree of genetic similarity (shared genetic interest) between individuals. Rudimentary forms of reciprocity can even arise in unrelated individuals without costly higher cognitive abilities through small evolutionary steps, but even then some means of monitoring personal state variables and for tracking the outcomes of prior interactions with others are necessary (Barta, McNamara, Huszar, & Taborsky, 2010). In humans, kin selection (reciprocity with genetically related people) may have served as the initial mechanism for the existence of reciprocity with genetically unrelated people. But it was then extended to unrelated individuals provided certain conditions exist, including those mentioned above (evaluating state variables and tracking prior interactional outcomes) (Barta et al., 2010; Cosmides & Tooby, 1992; Michod, 1999; Reeve, 1998).

The instrumental level of EF and its components play a role in bringing about the two conditions above needed to support reciprocity among unrelated individuals, including self-awareness of state and a mechanism for tracking prior interactional outcomes. A third condition is that there must be a greater payoff to both parties, either now or later, than would exist if either acted alone. Among kin, the payoff for reciprocity is an increase in genetic or inclusive fitness; it alone can explain the development of even unconscious, automatic altruistic and reciprocal behavior among genetically related individuals as seen across many species. There is no need for the individual to foresee the likely increased payoffs for reciprocating.

Foresight is a fourth condition. Among people who are not relatives, reciprocating requires foresight of a greater payoff than if one acted alone. It might be access to greater resources, breeding opportunities, or chances of increased survival. The payoff must not only be possible, it must be capable of being learned or foreseen based on past such encounters. The nonverbal working memory or visual imagery (ideational) component of EF provides just such a capacity for foresight. As that capacity expands and the time horizon over which the individual can contemplate outcomes increases into the possible future, the individual can conceive that longer-term self-interests are likely to converge with those of others. Recognition of that likelihood drives the willingness or motivation of individuals to reciprocate. The conception of longer-term mutual self-advantage creates the opportunity for and basis of social exchange.

A fifth condition applies in instances of delayed reciprocity where the payoff is to occur at a later time—there must be some means of accounting and recalling the conditions of the original exchange (Barta et al., 2010). Visual imagery and the hindsight it accords, I believe, provide just such a mental bookkeeping device for people, which was greatly boosted by external forms of recordkeeping (Barkley, 2001).

A further condition is that individuals must have some means of distinguishing a likely mutual reciprocator from a likely cheater or social parasite. Given that humans reciprocate frequently, we can expect them to possess some cognitive mechanism for assessing another person by facial expressions, postures, emotional signs, and other perceptual means (Cosmides & Tooby, 1992). But such judgments can be greatly facilitated by observational learning—watching what people do with each other and being inclined to reciprocate with those observed to engage honestly in this practice with others (Reeve, 1998). At the previous level of EF, visual imagery and its more general ideational capacity gave rise to vicarious learning. Where observational learning exists within groups, there is an opportunity for individuals to acquire reputations as reciprocators or cheaters because everyone can observe and recall everyone else's past behavior. Social reputations for trustworthiness can develop that signal the likelihood of successful reciprocation with that person in the future.

Several other conditions must also exist, however. One is that the individuals must be highly likely to encounter each other again, sometimes referred to as a low dispersal rate. This condition is afforded by group living. There also must be a means for reducing or addressing potential conflicts of self-interests that can arise by chance and not as intentional cheating. That mechanism is compromising.

A final condition is that there must be a physical or social cost to cheaters when their cheating has been detected. They must be punished within the group. Mechanisms for policing actions and for dispensing punishment are essential if reciprocity is to arise among unrelated individuals living in groups. In people, this willingness to dispense punishment to cheaters is likely part of the cultural background and determines even the likelihood of reciprocity arising between people (Gachter, Herrmann, & Thoni, 2010). To summarize, the conditions that give rise to reciprocity include hindsight and foresight, presence of kin, repeated encounters in group living, observational learning, and means of policing and punishing defectors or cheaters. Where such conditions are found to exist, reciprocity can arise and become a stable (enduring) strategy within the group (Axelrod, 1997; Reeve, 1998).

Because human groups include genetically related and unrelated individuals, they have the added adaptive advantage of a broader risk pool than would be the case among just genetically related people, as in families. That expansion of the risk pool is achieved by the opportunity to enter into acts of reciprocal exchange of goods and services with many other individuals regardless of genetic relationship. It provides a greater means of mutual survival than can just acts of reciprocity among kin. Social exchange acts like an insurance risk pool—individuals join the pool and contribute resources to it with the promise that the pooled resources will be shared with them should they have a need for a withdrawal. Risk pools are quite valuable when there are wide, often unpredictable fluctuations in resource availability and variability in human talent (Barkley, 2001). Those who succeed at acquiring more of a resource than is needed at the moment may exchange that bounty with another in need of it. But that is done with the understanding that a debt has now been incurred. That debt must be repaid in assets of at least equal value or repaid later in assets of equal or even greater value, that is, with interest. Interest on debt arises as a result of the time lag to the repayment and hence the loss of opportunity the lender has to use that resource during the period of indebtedness (Mises, 1990). It also arises because of the discounting of delayed consequences described in Chapter 4. Delayed repayments are less valuable to an individual for the same reason that delayed consequences are less valuable—the time lag to get them.

Visual Imagery (Hindsight) as the Bookkeeping Mechanism Needed for Reciprocity

Visual imagery and the conscious re-sensing of the past (hindsight) appear ideally suited to provide an accounting mechanism for tracking exchanges and activities with others. They also provide a basis for evaluating the benefits of cooperating with another (foresight). An ideal candidate for these mechanisms is the nonverbal working memory system, or what has been described in this model as sensing (or re-sensing) to the self. This is not merely speculative. Others have argued that nonverbal working memory is important in the development of social and emotional human activities (Rossano, 2010, 2011), and it has been shown to be so in the social interactions of young children (Ciairano et al., 2007). Moreover, deficits in working memory are associated with significant social impairments in children with ADHD (Kofler et al., 2011). This capacity for using working memory as a basis for social reciprocity and later cooperation is markedly enhanced by self-directed speech that adds symbolic guidance toward goals to sensory perceptual ones.

One prediction that arises from this line of argument is that visual imagery is likely to be present in other species that live in groups with others of limited or no genetic relationship and who engage in reciprocity and cooperation (chimpanzees and dolphins come to mind). Moreover, given the importance of these human social activities to survival, it is not surprising that this EF would begin its development exceptionally early. Hence self-awareness, inhibition, and visual–spatial imagery are likely to be the initial EFs at the Instrumental level that probably coevolved in human evolutionary history (phylogeny) and co-develop in individual human maturation (ontogeny) as noted previously.

EF, Reciprocity, and Economics

Humans cannot do two things at once. They must evaluate, prioritize, and choose their course of action. They must choose quickly and efficiently, for their life (time) is limited. And they must consider the impact of their choices on the other self-regulating goal-directed agents around them. Given these premises, people must make rapid cost-benefit calculations concerning their actions both now and over the longer term—this is the basis of the field of economics and human praxeology (Mises, 1990). Every choice and action involves a calculation of the costs and benefits for the individual. The inventions of money, arithmetic, and even double entry bookkeeping (cultural scaffolding) permitted a much quicker means for calculating such cost-benefit ratios for humans, particularly as they go about exchanging resources with others. Perhaps this is why most people think of economics as involving monetary calculations. But at its root, economics is about the making of choices among alternative means and ends. Defined in this way, economics pervades nearly every domain of major life activities. Each domain involves the need to choose and to act as seen in education, occupational functioning, social relations, money management, health maintenance, driving, cohabiting, child-rearing, or even having sex and reproducing. This is why EF is so pervasive in human life and so devastating when compromised. EF comprises those mental mechanisms humans use to make choices and initiate actions toward goals, and such choices are nearly universal in human action.

The components of EF are essential in directing and sustaining human action toward a goal. Self-awareness provides a person with a sense of their current state. Visual imagery and self-directed sensory–motor action provide the means for imagining a future state of less uneasiness or greater satisfaction. The difference between the current state and future state gives rise to the self-motivation to plan and act. The plan arises out of hindsight, self-directed speech, and the reconstitutional function of self-directed mental play. Enactment of the plan creates purposeful action. Such foresight, choice, and the calculated actions to which they lead are therefore the starting point for the study of economics.

Once the mechanism of reciprocity and its benefits are discovered through foresight and experience, the person enters a rudimentary level of the field of economics—social exchange. This is how EF/SR is linked to one of the most pervasive and uniquely human activities—economic behavior involving the use of others. An exchange of goods or services between two people *de facto* creates a protomarket. When done repeatedly between these individuals or among more people than this, it begins to form a market. Extended to human groups involving multiple such acts of reciprocity daily creates an economic system, or multiple processes of exchange. The location for such market exchanges eventually may become a common, specific setting or place, then known as a marketplace, but this should not disguise the fact that a market is a process, not a location (Mises, 1990). In such markets (processes), humans incur debts, barter and engage in other purchasing activity, and track and monitor these exchanges (via accounting) as they occur with multiple members of the group. Markets are therefore self-organizing among individuals with a sufficient level of EF development that supports the conception of the mutual longer-term benefits that can arise from the exchange. Markets are likely to be impossible or unstable when efforts to control them are imposed from outside the participants to this reciprocal exchange, especially under the conditions of coercion and authority. That is because those others cannot have access to the Instrumental or cognitive (private) EF level of each party to that exchange that subjectively values its benefits—the very basis for the exchange between them. Only the individual knows the value he or she assigns to the possible outcomes of the exchange, and so only they are the one capable of determining whether or not the exchange should take place and what or how much to exchange. Eventually, participants in the market (processes) may develop a set of mutually agreed upon rules for such participation (laws and contracts), a means for resolving conflicts among well-intentioned participants (mediation), and a means for punishing cheaters or parasites to the exchange (civil courts and police), thereby creating a more formal organization to the market based on cultural scaffolding. There must be a mental mechanism or set of mechanisms that permits and supports this type of subjective use calculation and such self-organized social exchanges or markets. Here I argue that it is the EF system, especially its capacity for forethought and culture, and its larger phenotype extended out to this Tactical–Reciprocal level.

Reciprocity, Morality, and Ethics

Daily human social life affords opportunities for sharing, taking turns, keeping promises, etiquette, repaying favors, and so on. Morality involves the self-regulation necessary to resist immediate urges, conform to social norms, defer to legitimate authorities, care for others, and essentially understand why certain acts are right or wrong (Krebs, 1998). To behave morally, individuals must subordinate their immediate short-term self-interests to those of another while expecting to receive similar treatment the next time when the situation is reversed. Psychologists would therefore consider reciprocity and self-subordination (self-restraint) as important social practices in cultivating and sustaining relationships. Yet psychology has traditionally viewed the origins of morality as arising from the social environment and the early training of children by parents, whether through frustrating early instinctual desires as in psychoanalysis or through observational learning. Evolutionary psychology, however, has shown that other species have evolved prototypical forms of morality such as reciprocity. It is therefore possible to explain human morality, at least in part, as arising out of biological evolution as seen in other social species. Morality would also be predicted from Game Theory when applied to the long-term interests of two essentially self-interested beings (Hauser, 2006; Krebs, 1998; Ridley, Matt, 1997; Wright, 1994). In short, it is not always in the best interests of a self-interested creature to always maximize short-term interests; it is possible to derive a greater payoff by reciprocating on some occasions with others. Krebs (1998) explains why:

> The unconstrained pursuit of individual interests and the exploitation of others are ineffective interpersonal strategies for three main reasons. First, some resources are beyond the reach of individuals acting alone. Second, unconstrained selfishness may destroy the system of cooperation on which it feeds. Third, others are evolved to resist being exploited. In effect, individuals in cooperative groups agree to adopt moral strategies of interaction to maximize their mutual gain, although not necessarily consciously or explicitly. Moral rules uphold these strategies, defining the investments (e.g. duties) each individual is expected to make to obtain the returns (e.g. rights). (1998, p. 339)

The evolutionary foundation for morality, therefore, may be reciprocity among individuals who live in close proximity and frequently encounter each other while pursuing their respective self-interests. The capacity to consciously evaluate self-interests over longer terms could easily have further boosted the push that evolution may give into the path of behaving reciprocally and hence morally. I will return to this point shortly.

When humans live in groups and repeatedly intersect with each other as they each pursue their own goals, there is also the repeated likelihood that their paths and goals will conflict. Such potential for conflict creates a need for "rules of the road" to make such interactions progress more smoothly or peacefully. There is, therefore, a need for the development of ethics, or at least protoethics, at this level of EF. Ethics are the rules or principles that people adopt for pursuing their goals (values) in the context of other self-interested goal-directed people. Ethics provide rules that have been learned over time to facilitate peaceful group living and to lessen the inevitable potential for conflicts among varying self-interests that arise in that mode of living. By adopting and following an ethical rule, individuals are more likely to attain their goals while not interfering with others who are doing so. Ethics thereby facilitates peaceful coexistence as each pursues his or her own goals and strives to maximize his or her own welfare and happiness. In short, ethics exist because they reduce human conflict. Such rules are necessary if one wishes to encourage the likelihood of future interactions and exchanges with each other.

Ethics are like the rules we adopt for driving so that all drivers can get to their destinations more efficiently and effectively while interacting with other drivers. They are the rules of the road for human social interactions if one expects to pursue one's self-interests with as little conflict with others as possible and to increase the likelihood of future exchanges with others. Ethical rules can also be one means that facilitate individuals' ability to subordinate their short-term, smaller, or less urgent self-interests for the sake of attaining longer-term, larger, or more urgent ones through reciprocity with others. The Golden Rule is a classic example of just such an ethic.

The foregoing argument clearly links the actions of reciprocity (and cooperation, to be discussed in Chapter 7) to a need for and basis of ethics. How then do we link ethics back even further to EF? Allow me to let Hazlitt (1998) do it in his own words, recalling that the term "desire" is another word for wants, ends, or goals—the difference between our current state of dissatisfaction or uneasiness and an imagined future state of greater satisfaction:

> How, then, do we move from any basis of desire to any theory of ethics?
> We find the solution when we take a longer and broader view. All of our desires may be generalized desires to substitute a more satisfactory state of affairs for a less satisfactory state. It is true that an individual, under the immediate influence of impulse or passion, or the desire for revenge, or gluttony, or an overwhelming craving for a release of sexual tension, or for a smoke or a drink or a drug, may in the long run only reduce a more satisfactory state to a less satisfactory state, may make himself less happy rather than more happy. But this less satisfactory state was not his real conscious intention even at the moment of the acting. He realizes, in retrospect, that this action was folly; he did not improve his condition, but made it worse; he did not act in accordance with his long-run interests, but against them. He is always willing to recognize, in his calmer moments, that he should choose the action that best promotes his own interests and maximizes his own happiness (or minimizes his own unhappiness) *in the long run*. Wise

and disciplined men refuse to indulge in immediate pleasures when the indulgence seems only too likely to lead in the long run to an overbalance of misery or pain.

. . . Mankind has found, over the centuries, that certain rules of action best tend to promote the long-run happiness of both the individual and society. These rules of action have come to be called *moral* rules. Therefore, assuming that one seeks one's long-run happiness, these are the rules one *ought* to follow.

Certainly, this is the whole basis of what is called *prudential* ethics. In fact, wisdom, or the art of living wisely, is perhaps only another name for prudential ethics. (pp. 12–13; emphasis in original)

Note that the core of ethics is the individual's capacity to contemplate his or her own welfare *over the long-term*, a capacity as noted earlier that arose from the Instrumental level of EF (foresight) and was just as essential a condition for reciprocity (social exchange) and as the starting point of economics. It includes a capacity to contemplate the welfare of or consequences to others as well as one's self as a result of the actions and goals being contemplated. Moral dilemmas arise, in fact, when such longer-term self-interests of one individual or the means they are using to pursue them work at cross purposes to those of another. Research indicates that the PFC and hence the EF system participates in a person's efforts to confront and resolve just such moral dilemmas (Hauser, 2006; Wright, 1994).

To reiterate, EF/SR extends outward as a phenotype to become essential to social exchange (reciprocity) and trading, as well as to ethics and economics. That is because it provides the means by which (1) we perceive and conceive of the future or the longer term and so of the greater payoffs that these social activities can provide to us; (2) we are able to construct and follow rules to guide our choices and commensurate actions over that time period; (3) we rapidly calculate the costs-benefits (subjective value) of those choices (means and ends) over time beforehand; (4) we restrain or otherwise subordinate our immediate short-term interests to our longer-term interests so as to obtain greater mediate or longer-term consequences; (5) we activate, manage, and otherwise regulate emotional and motivational states in the service of these goals in the context of the actions and motivations of others; and (6) we self-organize the environment and others within it so as to be more likely to attain our goals and to attain larger goals than by acting in isolation, independently, or parasitically. This makes plain the outward extension of the Instrumental level of the EF phenotype through human action up through the Self-Reliant level and then on outward further to this Reciprocal one.

Using Each Other for Mutual Self-Regulation

Social relationships also can be used to boost an individual's EF/SR (Finkel & Fitzsimons, 2011). This is especially the case in cohabiting or other intimate relationships, and it may even be found in occupational settings that involve reciprocity or social exchange. The relationship of EF/SR to social relations may also be bidirectional. An individual's degree of EF/SR may positively or adversely affect their social relations with others (Fitzsimons & Finkel, 2011), while those others may interact with us in a way that increases or decreases our own likelihood of SR and goal attainment (Finkel & Fitzsimons, 2011). As Carver and Scheier (2011) noted, self-regulation (or EF) can be thought of as a four-step process in which one engages in *goal setting and initiation* (goal choice), *goal operation* (the course of action being pursued toward the goal), *goal monitoring* (feedback on the current state relative to the desired goal), and *effective outputs* (using the feedback to adjust actions, rate of progress, and even to reprioritize goals). Each of these steps can be reciprocally facilitated or impeded by one's social relationships, especially those with parents or intimate partners (Finkel & Fitzsimons, 2011). The important point here is that the EF/SR phenotype now extends outward to create social effects at a distance and to use those social influences to boost one's EF/SR effectiveness in attaining one's goals.

The Sociometer in the Extended EF Phenotype

People appear to possess a mental mechanism for monitoring their moment-to-moment status within a social group. This mechanism picks up social signals pertinent to appraising one's own relational value to others. This value can be captured along a dimension of acceptance–rejection. A proto-sociometer may, in fact, exist in some form at the Pre-Executive level in social species such as ourselves. What emerges at this Tactical–Reciprocal level of EF/SR is that individuals are consciously aware of the results of this evaluative module and the emotions it generates. As a result, they can also consciously intervene in or even override the process. EF can be used to govern the sociometer in a manner similar to how it governs the more automatic level of human behavior described in Chapter 3. Recall that there is a primary emotional module at the Pre-Executive level and a secondary emotion-regulating (EF) module that arises from self-awareness of emotions. The EF level can consciously intervene in the primary emotional process to self-regulate those emotions. So, too, one can intervene to self-regulate one's relational value to others.

If signals of social dislike or rejection are detected, corrective action can be consciously implemented. Or such signals can be consciously overridden by reappraisal of the situational context and the initial feelings it engenders. One's self-esteem appears to be a by-product of this sociometer (Leary & Guadagno, 2011). Other new EF components may arise here as well, but this makes the point that not all EF components may be apparent at the instrumental cognitive level being evaluated solely by traditional psychometric EF tests.

Understanding EF at this Tactical–Reciprocal level captures what is often lost, with near tragic consequences, in individuals with severe PFC injuries, as noted in numerous accounts dating back to even the earliest descriptions of such patients. It characterizes the far-reaching adverse qualitative social changes that take place in injured patients' behavior as a consequence (i.e., Phineas Gage; Harlow, 1848, 1868). Despite the plethora of descriptions of the social disabilities often experienced by patients with PFC damage and hence EF deficits (Luria, 1966; Stuss & Benson, 1986), the traditional assessment of EF by cognitive tests misses these social levels of analysis completely.

The Role of Parenting and Culture in Reciprocity

This model of EF has been developed only recently, and so sufficient research does not exist on the developmental course and sequencing of these EF levels as they emerge in childhood. Nevertheless, it seems sensible that EF tactics may initially emerge in children as a means to artificially arranged ends constructed by parents or other adults. Their purpose is to develop social skills, rule following, and reciprocity of social interactions, such as sharing, turn-taking, reciprocal exchange, and even altruism, especially to move children up to not only the Self-Reliant level of EF but further upward to its Reciprocal level. An example is pliance training for rule-following. Parents provide an artificial consequence to young children for why their social rule is to be obeyed (Hayes et al., 1996). Such artificial consequences are eventually withdrawn once the delayed natural consequences from such rule-following arise to maintain the rule-governed behavior (Hayes, 1989). Similar forms of parent and later teacher scaffolding may be provided for children around the tactics of self-management to time intervals, self-organization, self-motivation, and self-regulation of emotions. This social scaffolding can eventually be withdrawn (dismantled) as the child's abilities develop further and as these activities are eventually maintained by their natural social (and other) consequences, assisted by the child's greater capacity for hindsight and foresight over longer time periods.

EF tactics in children may therefore initially be a means to immediate or near-term ends, both artificially arranged by others and naturally occurring. Parents and teachers may understand the longer-term goal that each tactic is in the service of achieving. But to the child the socially arranged consequences of adults are the ends in themselves until the longer-term consequences for employing such tactics occur.

Culture also provides other scaffolding at this level, such as written rules, laws, policing, formal contracts, and other conditions that may be required for such reciprocity and exchange. Such contracts are unnecessary when one buys things such as relatively low-value items at a store. But contracts may become necessary when the exchange involves greater values or takes place over a considerable delay, as when purchasing a home. Reading, writing, and arithmetic are cultural artifacts passed along to each generation to facilitate social reciprocity or exchanges. They are not instinctive or inborn, but like many such cultural devices, they must be learned. Once learned, they and many other cultural devices ratchet upward the person's ability to pursue goals through reciprocity.

Implications for EF Tests

The foregoing line of reasoning implies that, with development, the social environment has a growing impact on EF/SR effectiveness that would not be detected if only the cognitive (Instrumental) level of EF is assessed. It also supports the stance taken here that the EF system exists largely to address social purposes. It should now be evident why tests of the Instrumental, moment-to-moment, nonsocial, cognitive level of EF processes are not strongly related to EF assessments at the day-to-day level of social interaction. First, the spans of time over which such behavior must be planned and organized are dramatically different. Instrumental EFs are assessed over minutes of time, while tactical EFs must cope with social events lasting hours to days or even to weeks. The Instrumental level of EF is to the Tactical level what a few minutes is to a day or a week. The former is a severely limited ascertainment window over which to observe EF play out in human affairs. Cross-temporal awareness, organization, and maintenance of goal-directed action with problem solving requires a time horizon of considerably longer range than in a clinical testing appointment. The individual must comprehend, evaluate, and even anticipate social events. This will play out markedly further ahead in time than that represented at the Instrumental level of just minutes to a few hours.

New EF components likely come into play here at the Tactical–Reciprocal level that are not represented (or at least not usually assessed) at the Instrumental level. Just as modules for theory of mind and mirror–neuron modules for imitation/vicarious learning arose at the last level to assist EF/SR, new modules would need to arise at this level that were not present at lower ones. These include learning rules pertinent to social skills such as rules of etiquette, subordinating immediate self-interests to one's longer-term interests, and rules for reciprocity (sharing, turn-taking, promise keeping, trading, and repaying). It may also include mental mechanisms useful to assessing one's relational value to others, a mental device called the sociometer (Leary & Guadagno, 2011).

Conclusions

This level of the extended EF phenotype allows us to amend the definition of EF as follows: *the use of self-directed actions so as to choose goals and to select, enact, and sustain actions across time toward those goals usually in the context of others **often relying on social means.*** In this instance, that social means is reciprocity—mutual exchange of resources, goods, and services that yields a greater longer-term payoff for participants than had either party acted alone or tried to parasitize the other.

This level of EF can be characterized by the increases in the eight developmental capacities that are derived from EF and that are needed to attain this level. The Tactical–Reciprocal level is portrayed graphically in Figure 6.1. The extended EF phenotype is shown as a series of concentric rings now including this new level. The rings are labeled, and the labels reflect the levels' stepped hierarchy. The eight capacities have changed as follows:

1. Environmental *spatial* contemplation and self-organization expands from rearrangement of the physical, proximal environment to a greater distance from the individual.
2. The time horizon or *temporal* window for contemplation must expand to days and weeks to reveal the longer-term benefits of social reciprocity.

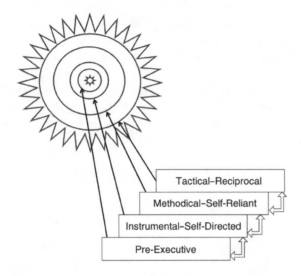

FIGURE 6.1. Two different ways of illustrating the extended EF phenotype as it occurs at the Tactical–Reciprocal level. The concentric rings at the left indicate the outwardly radiating nature of the phenotype at this intermediate stage of development (Pre-Executive, Instrumental–Self-Directed, Methodical–Self-Reliant, Tactical–Reciprocal). The stacked boxes at the lower right indicate the hierarchical arrangement of these four phenotypic levels. The bidirectional arrows to the right of each box are intended to convey the bidirectional flow of information between the levels. Information from the lower levels flows upward to the higher levels, while management of the lower levels may be exerted downward by the next higher level.

3. The needed degree of *inhibition* and self-restraint is greater than that needed for social self-defense seen at the last level. Moral and ethical rules require individuals to subordinate their immediate, short-term self-interests to those of others as well as to their own longer-term welfare.

4. With these expansions come increasing valuation and *motivation* for further delayed consequences than was evident at earlier levels.

5. The level of *abstract* rules and concepts is considerably higher as social rules must be understood and adopted to facilitate reciprocity, including such rules as social skills, ethics, and laws.

6. The level of *behavioral* complexity needed within this zone is moderate; it is far greater than that needed in lower levels of EF but not as complex as that seen in the next level.

7. The need for and complexity of *social* interactions is moderate; the individual is now pursuing goals using reciprocity and social exchange.

8. The bidirectional influence of *culture* has increased as individuals not only absorb cultural practices and use cultural devices for their own goal-directed activities, but they may now contribute new cultural products and devices to the culture via reciprocity and trade.

7

The Strategic–Cooperative Level

The dividing line between the Tactical–Reciprocal and Strategic–Cooperative levels is not as distinct as that between lower levels. The transition upward to this new level most likely occurs when several conditions come to exist. First, the individual's capacity to take a longer-term view concerning goals and consequences expands even further than at the previous EF level. Second, as a consequence of having moved up to the previous EF level, individuals find that they are interacting more often in mutually beneficial ways with many others. They may find themselves living in closer proximity to others or near marketplaces. Low rates of dispersal (group living) and frequent mutually beneficial interactions set the stage for contemplating an even higher level of social organization—the principle that people working together as a group can accomplish more than any of them working alone or through mere reciprocity. Acting cooperatively presupposes a shared or common interest that each cooperator can understand and use to calculate the risks and benefits to cooperation (Brown & Vincent, 2008). Third, the individual finds that EF tactics being employed for a goal can become a submeans to attain larger, longer-term ones. Sets of tactics are required to bridge the longer delay to the later goal. A strategy is a set of tactics for the attainment of a longer-term, higher-order goal than is possible with a tactic alone. When such nested sets of tactics are required for a larger end, the strategic level has been attained. Just as there is a hierarchical structure to the programming of behavioral sequences and even nested sets of sequences from the posterior to the anterior aspects of the PFC (Badre, 2008; Botvinich, 2008), so too is there a hierarchical arrangement to the extended phenotype of EF from Instrumental to Methodical to Tactical to this Strategic level.

Generally, I believe that the Tactical and Strategic levels of EF eventually become distinguished as a consequence of (1) a growing awareness of longer spatial distances and spans of time that result in the lengthening of the space–time horizon over which actions, goals, and consequences are being contemplated; (2) the commensurate increase in the magnitude of the values, desires, wants, and goals (consequences) being pursued; (3) the increasingly lengthy and more complex hierarchical structure of the behavioral sets, nested sets, and their sequences necessary to attain such long-term goals; (4) the use of more general, abstract, and universal rules for planning and guiding behavior toward goals; (5) the growing complexity of the social network likely to be needed for coordinated action or cooperation and not needed merely for social reciprocity and exchange; and (6) the greater reliance on and invention of culture as social scaffolding for further boosting EF/SR. All of these factors arise out of the further maturation of the PFC, the developmental capacities initially granted by the evolution of EF, and the sociocultural scaffolding that has been inherited from prior generations. In concert, they lead to the emergence of this higher, more behaviorally and socially complex, and longer-term level of EF. Other conditions for cooperative living must also exist for it to be a stable strategy, as discussed below, but these are sufficient to at least cause the individual to contemplate the opportunities for him or her that are inherent in group action as a unit.

The Advent of Social Cooperation in the Extended EF Phenotype

When relatively long-lived individuals live in groups and have low dispersal rates, they will have opportunities to form coalitions with others in pursuit of the same goal. A group of individuals acting in unison, or as a single unit, to achieve a shared or common goal, have formed "a cooperative." It is not just going along with a request of another or getting along with other people without conflict. The specific meaning of a cooperative as used here is a group enterprise to achieve a shared goal. Cooperatives allow individuals of like-minded self-interest to accomplish much larger goals than can be done alone. By doing so each gains additional resources or benefits that none could gain individually or through reciprocal exchange. Reciprocity constituted zero-sum interactions, with no gain in total value from the exchange. Acting cooperatively as a group creates opportunities for nonzero-sum interactions (Wright, 2000). Such interactions are characterized by a net increase in total values or assets across all participating parties (Kelly, 2010; Mises, 1990; Ridley, Matt, 2010). Group hunting and foraging are examples. Such cooperative activities may form only around the accomplishment of a common goal, then dissolve and re-form with other members around other shared goals. The duration of the particular cooperatives depends in part on the time period over which the goal must be pursued by the cooperative. Its size is determined in part by the magnitude of the goal being contemplated and the number of individuals required to achieve it.

EF has been shown to be an important contributor to cooperative social behavior in children (Best et al., 2009; Ciariano et al., 2007; Mischel et al., 1989; Mischel, Shoda, & Rodriguez, 1989). It is also evident over early development in the substantial inverse relationship between increases in degree of self-control (EF) and decreases in social deviance and antisocial conduct; the variance shared between these two trajectories may be as high as 75% (Vazsonyi & Huang, 2010). Moreover, it is also a serious deficit in individuals with significant injuries to the EF/PFC system (Harlow, 1848; Luria, 1966; Stuss & Benson, 1986).

The Strategic–Cooperative level of EF emerges over a considerably longer period of human development than earlier levels and requires that those earlier levels be attained before it can emerge. Whereas reciprocity typically involves relatively short social interactions of exchange, cooperation requires concerted action over a longer time frame. Acting as a cooperative or unified group having a shared goal is also more complex than dyadic social interactions that exist in reciprocal exchanges. Cooperatives require a higher level of cognitive EF development to contemplate, organize, initiate, and sustain, yet they give rise to a greater payoff. While reciprocity among unrelated individuals is relatively rare in the living world, cooperative group action among such organisms is an even rarer event.

The extended phenotype of EF can now be diagrammed as follows:

CNS pre-executive functions → CNS executive (self-self-regulatory)
functions → executive (self-regulatory) adaptive behavior →
self-organization of environmental arrangements (methods, products,
artifacts) → self-organizing of reciprocal exchanges with others →
organization of cooperative ventures with a group

Cooperative action is not only evident in humans. It has arisen multiple times at significant transitions in biological evolution as when genes combined to create chromosomes, cells combined to create eukaryotes, eukaryotic cells combined to create multicellular bodies, and when those individual bodies combine to create a social cooperative (Maynard Smith & Szathmary, 1999; Michod, 1999). However, all of these instances of cooperation can arise when the entities have a high degree of genetic similarity and it is in their genetic self-interests. The greater payoff in these cases is an increase in inclusive fitness, the likelihood of getting one's genes into the next generation. This serves to explain why cooperation in humans, when it does arise, does so most often among genetically related family members. That is not the case when humans form a cooperative with others who are not genetic relatives.

Conditions Necessary for Cooperation to Arise

For a cooperative to exist at any of the major evolutionary transitions, certain conditions had to exist that made such cooperatives more beneficial to the participating individual's self-interests than would pursuit of those self-interests in isolation or even with exchange. Cooperative formation requires a transfer of some of the benefits of the lower levels of independent action and of reciprocity to that of the cooperating group and its actions (Michod, 1999). This is likely to be as true of human consciously formed cooperatives as it is of all earlier forms of evolved cooperation.

The conditions for the formation of a cooperative are largely the same ones necessary for reciprocity to occur among unrelated people as discussed in the last chapter. To reiterate, these requirements are (from Michod, 1999): (1) a low rate of dispersal (people must live in close proximity); (2) a capacity for a greater payoff for cooperative formation over time than from self-reliance or reciprocity (Brown & Vincent, 2008); (3) a means of keeping track of everyone's individual contributions to the cooperative venture and hence their share of the goal (bookkeeping); (4) a way of reducing conflict, such as compromising in human interactions; and (5) a means of policing the participants' activities to detect and punish cheaters or free riders. To these conditions, three additional ones must now be added that were unnecessary for reciprocity: (6) a means of encouraging or even coercing group participants to join in that punitive activity (Gachter & Herrmann, 2009); (7) a high degree of perceived similar self-interest (Leimar & Hammerstein, 2010; Michod, 1999), including similarity of phenotype (Antal, Ohtsuki, Wakeley, Taylor, & Nowak, 2009); and (8) a means of reducing individual differences in unshared self-interests (Axelrod, 1997; Michod, 1999). In short, punishment must be dispensed by the cooperative to its cheating individual members (Barta et al., 2010; Fehr & Gachter, 2000; Fehr & Schmidt, 1999; Gachter et al., 2010), shared self-interests must be high or enhanced (Leimar & Hammerstein, 2010), and dissimilarities must be low or minimized (Michod, 1999). Where such preconditions do not exist, the cooperative venture is unlikely to arise, or if it has, it is likely to deteriorate and dissolve. This may account for why some of the earliest forms of human cooperative action arose within genetically related families. Under that circumstance, these conditions are the most likely to exist. In humans, it is the capacity to foresee the longer-term greater personal benefits (expanded foresight) that is most important for cooperative action to arise among unrelated individuals. This probably accounts for the fact that cooperation among unrelated individuals is extremely unusual in the history of all organisms, because most species lack this capacity. Yet when cooperation does succeed, it affords participants a higher level of adaptive fitness and greater success in attaining their goals than could occur by individuals acting alone.

Cheating, free-riding, deceit, or fraud also arise as a possibility in such a cooperative enterprise, as in not contributing one's equal share of effort while obtaining an unfair share of the outcome. Mental mechanisms are therefore needed to detect cheaters. These may simply be elaborations of those that support reciprocal exchange (Cosmides & Tooby, 1992), as noted in Chapter 6. Yet there must also be a cultural background that provides sufficient opportunities to punish cheaters (increase the costs for cheating) (Brown & Vincent, 2008; Gachter & Herrmann, 2009; Gachter et al., 2010). However, there is a greater complexity and longer duration in cooperative ventures than in simpler dyadic interactions and exchanges with others. This necessitates a progression through the earlier EF levels in order to build up the earlier social relationships. That is to say, instrumental EF, self-reliance and self-defense, and reciprocity are prerequisites to the formation of a cooperative social group.

Cooperative action, as noted above, means not just reciprocity but action often taken in unison for shared self-interest. An example is when several farmers join together to move boulders off of an individual's farmland. Without machines, this goal is difficult to achieve by acting alone; and all farmers in the cooperative can benefit as long as all agree to do this for each farmer's land. The same is true if they join together to build each other houses or barns or to aid each other in harvesting crops in as timely a manner as possible to avoid spoilage. Joint cooperative action accomplishes goals none can achieve alone or achieve as quickly or efficiently. Such cooperative activities fall under the rubric of the Strategic–Cooperative level of EF.

It is very possible that new mental modules may be needed at this level of EF. For instance, new mental abilities may be needed here to boost the ethics and associated morality that arose at the level of reciprocity. The psychological capacities for the social emotions of conscience, sympathy, empathy, guilt, remorse, and a sense of belonging with others may have arisen as a consequence of social cooperation and to further facilitate its occurrence. Under such conditions, it is also possible for certain individuals to exist who are good at faking such important signals so as to hijack cooperative ventures for their own immediate self-interests (selfishness), as in psychopathy or sociopathy.

Where cooperatives exist in nature and have done so for exceptionally long periods, it may become increasingly difficult, if not impossible, for the evolutionary sequence to reverse itself with a return to isolated or reciprocal activity. For example, chromosomes are no longer likely to break apart to become individual genes again, complex eukaryotic cells are not likely to break apart to return to the formerly prokaryotic state, nor are multicelled bodies likely to break apart and disperse as single-celled organisms again. That is because one by-product of cooperative activity is that the participating individuals lose some of the adaptive features that were essential to their earlier solitary survival. Because the features needed at earlier stages are no longer required, they atrophy or eventually fail to develop at all (Maynard Smith & Szathmary, 1999). This arises because of a special feature of cooperatives not evident in self-reliance or reciprocity—a division of labor, or specialization of function. It is far more efficient and cost-effective for individuals to relinquish their redundant and hence inefficient features and to specialize within the cooperative venture.

The Importance of Division of Labor to a Cooperative

Biological evolution has repeatedly discovered the advantages of division of labor within a cooperative, whether between genes that form chromosomes or specialized cells and organs that form bodies. Division of labor must have offered advantages to all participants, given its repeated occurrence in evolutionary history. As with the evolution of biological cooperatives, special conditions had to exist for the division of labor to evolve in human cooperatives. In the case of genes, cells, and families, it is shared genetic self-interest plus one additional ingredient: natural variation in abilities.

Nature is always unequal in the distribution of talents. Individual variability in talent comes into existence because of genetic variability. Inequality also comes into play in the uneven distribution of environmental resources across regions. Both genetics and environment are unfair and uneven in the manner in which they influence the development of any given individual. That variability is the source for the benefits of a division of labor. If all were equally talented, little benefit would be had by forming a long-term cooperative using division of labor. Self-reliance or even short-term concerted mutual effort among individuals might arise but beyond this there seems to be little benefit to forming a longer-term cooperative and dividing up labor based on abilities. But all are not equally talented in all things. Over time, as groups act in unison for shared goals, it will become evident that some are better at doing some things within the shared enterprise than are others. A time arises when it is worth considering having individual members of the group specialize in what they are best at doing.

How is division of labor within a cooperative more beneficial? As an example, consider that one individual may excel at making fishnets from vines or cord. But this person is a rather mediocre fisherman and even worse at either collecting the salt from the nearby salt marsh needed to preserve the catch or simply has been denied access to it by its current occupier. All three activities take time, but the individual is more efficient and skilled at net-making and thus able create more and better products in less time than he is at fishing or salt collecting. Another individual in the group excels at fishing, but she is poor at constructing a net and also not good at salt-collecting or, again, lacks the access to collect it. The occupier of the salt marsh in contrast is far better able to collect salt than to make nets or fish. Now all three people could continue to engage in all three activities and get by. But they are likely to achieve even better results if one concentrates more effort on net-making, another on fishing, and the third on salt-collecting and then exchange nets, fish, and salt among themselves in a cooperative. All are now far better off (have a greater net gain) than had they not formed a cooperative with division of labor in this fashion (Kelly, 2010; Mises, 1990; Ridley, Matt, 2010). But to achieve this advantage from this higher level of social organization, individuals must give up some things that they previously possessed or could do. They must sacrifice some self-interest in the short term to obtain greater personal benefits in the longer term. In doing so, they must become interdependent to such a degree that each is less able to succeed alone once the sacrifices have been made. The cooperative requires a level of commitment and trust not required of the individual who is entirely self-reliant or even those self-reliant people who engage in exchange of their excesses. A failure to cooperate at any link in this interdependent chain places all of its members at risk relative to those individuals who are solely self-reliant. But the benefits outweigh the risks. Done within a group, this type of division of labor with trading also creates a form of insurance that can smooth out wide swings in resource availability that may occur over time (see Kelly, 2010; Ridley, Matt, 2010, for examples). And it can do so better than can simple reciprocity. The three people have now formed an interdependent cooperative to everyone's mutual benefit. They have achieved a form of acting as a unitary entity similar to other types of acting in unison to achieve a common goal. While I fish, you make nets, and a third person collects salt and we meet up later to trade among ourselves. Each counts on and trusts the others to engage in their specialty while the others are simultaneously doing so, and all will trade their excess at a predetermined time, resulting in greater benefits to all than each could do alone.

Among humans, division of labor is a conscious, volitional, purposive activity and not just a by-product of evolution acting at the unconscious genetic level of self-interests or at an automatic level of behavior. Therefore, like reciprocity, it requires a special suite of mental mechanisms to permit the perception of both the principle of division of labor and its long-term mutual benefits, despite the initial self-sacrifice of shorter-term self-interests. That mechanism, once again, is foresight—a sense of the future.

Wherever they have been consciously discovered by human groups, the joint principles of cooperative group living (division of labor with trade) have led throughout human history to cultural and economic success and a higher quality of life (Kelly, 2010; Mises, 1990; Ridley, Matt, 2010). Division of labor boosts personal efficiency as well as productivity so that individuals can attain their goals more readily and have more time to pursue additional goals. Increases in efficiency and productivity contribute to a rise in the standard of living for all participating parties. This is an economic side of EF/SR that seems lost to researchers in the fields of neuropsychology, developmental psychology, and even personality and social psychology where studies of EF and SR have virtually ignored the essential involvement of EF/SR in human economic activity—a form of activity that pervades all human life (Mises, 1990).

The discovery of barter and trade between self-reliant individuals likely preceded the discovery and full-scale adoption of social cooperatives, and those likely preceded the further development of cooperatives based on division of labor and trade (Mises, 1990; Ridley, Matt, 2010). In the first situation (reciprocity), each person may be striving to be self-sufficient producing whatever they require for their survival and welfare by themselves (or as a family of mutually and genetically self-interested individuals). Yet they may transact a trade to obtain something of value that another has produced in excess of what that person needs. In the second situation, a cooperative may form around a single specific goal among otherwise self-reliant individuals, such as the cooperative boulder clearing mentioned earlier among self-reliant farmers living in relatively close proximity. Eventually individuals come to realize that they vary in their talents for doing things. Through foresight and reasoning this can lead them to understand that by each pursuing his or her talent more exclusively, the excess can be traded to other specialists within the cooperative. By this cooperative venture, a greater gain is obtained for each and all (Mises, 1990; Ridley, Matt, 2010).

The formation of a social cooperative that is founded on division of labor and trade appears to be the source of *sustained cooperation and community living* (Mises, 1990; Ridley, Matt, 2010). Recall that reciprocity involved trading one's excess goods or services to another. It was not mandatory but volitional and not a requirement for survival among self-reliant people. Under a social cooperative founded on division of labor, there is a need to trade because each has sacrificed some or all of their self-reliant abilities or activities to specialize and thus made themselves interdependent on the cooperative—things that did not happen with reciprocity among self-reliant people. Besides this sacrifice and the dependency on trade, a further consequence of the division of labor often necessitates that people live in closer proximity to each other because of the need for frequent trading. And they must do so peacefully if the added gains for all laborer/traders are to be realized over that which can arise from self-reliant people meeting periodically to exchange. If I am to make nets and yet obtain food to eat and preserve, I need to reside within a reasonable distance of the individual doing the fishing and the one harvesting the salt, both of whom are trading their excesses for the nets I have made. The more specialized is the division of labor, the closer individuals will have to reside in order to meet their respective needs and the greater the number of individuals needed to do so. Towns and cities spring up as a consequence.

To live in close proximity and engage in division of labor with trade, individuals in this social cooperative must subordinate some of their short-term desires and urges (sexual, aggressive, etc.) or risk losing others' cooperation and hence the capacity to gain from trade with them. These living arrangements create a need for a higher grade of ethics (how people should treat each other to sustain cooperative behavior) and laws (governing property rights and contracts) (Hazlitt, 1998; Mises, 1990) than were needed at the lower level of reciprocity.

The Profound Role of Culture in Cooperatives

The Cooperative level of the EF extended phenotype is greatly facilitated by culture—the inheritance of previous innovations that form scaffolding for further advancement and adaptive improvement of lower levels of EF. Language, myth, reading, writing, arithmetic, bookkeeping, ethics, laws, contracts, formal mechanisms for mediating disputes, police, courts, and group-sanctioned punishments of law violators are cultural inventions that arose out of EF and are applied at this level of the extended phenotype. As noted earlier, the likelihood of cooperation among people is partially dependent on the cultural background and the opportunities it affords for the policing and punishment of cheaters (Gachter & Herrmann, 2009; Gachter et al., 2010)—in other words, the costs and benefits it provides for cooperation versus cheating (Brown & Vincent, 2008). Cultural scaffolding is comprised not only of previously created products or artifacts, but also of other forms of information that pertain to beneficial rules for group organization that are passed along through verbally transmitted stories, myths, and folk wisdom, as well as more recent written records. The existence of culture means that each individual or cooperative does not have to start again from scratch to discover useful means to various goals. Standing on the cultural shoulders of all who came before, individuals can use the extant culture to be more efficient in their EF/SR pursuits toward their goals and contribute new innovations, products, services, records, and so on, that improve their own goal-pursuits and longer-term welfare while bettering the lives of others and subsequent generations. The transmission of culture is therefore both vertical (across generations), and horizontal (across existing people) (Durham, 1991). When the principles operating within cooperatives, division of labor with trade, and policing and punishment of cheaters, are combined with a cultural inheritance and the human EF of innovation (reconstitution), you get a cultural explosion of progress and development (Ridley, Matt, 2010); this explosion most likely launched early human societies and city-states 6,000 to 10,000 years ago.

As at earlier levels of EF/SR, individuals (and now groups) arrange external environmental, social, and cultural structures to amplify and facilitate cooperative activities. These structures are far more complex, abstract, and even longer-term rearrangements than at earlier levels. At this level, individuals organize cooperatives to facilitate the attainment of mutual goals or to boost individual benefits beyond what each individual can achieve alone or through simple exchange among self-reliant people. Nonetheless, these forms of self-organization also use the environment to facilitate goal-directed activities to further facilitate mutual benefits. Through such means we serve to regulate ourselves and each other for the greater gain of all parties to the cooperative enterprise.

This level also may represent more fully matured forms of EF discussed at the lower Tactical–Reciprocal level. For example, this Strategic–Cooperative level of EF may include EF abilities such as self-management across time, self-organization and problem solving, self-discipline, self-motivation, and self-regulation of emotions as employed over weeks, months, and even years to attain one's long-term goals and to see to one's longer-term welfare at these durations (Barkley, 2011a). Certainly, new strategies and cultural practices may develop that involve external means to support time management, self-organization, and problem solving, among other EF (EA) that emerged at the tactical level.

For instance, a small group of coworkers could form in order to monitor daily goal-directed performances, perhaps by meeting at the start of each day, over lunch, and at the end of the day. In each encounter, the group reviews each person's goals and evaluates progress so as to boost each person's successful self-regulation over time at the Strategic level of EF. Certainly, where work assignments have been given to the entire group or team, then such activities become essential. Making one's self publicly accountable to others for behavior change and ongoing self-regulation is itself a strategy at this level of EF. Thus, arranging the larger social and nonsocial environment to further support the initiation and maintenance of self-regulation toward goals over time represents EF strategies that can be translated into shorter term daily to weekly tactics to facilitate successful goal attainment over longer terms.

This level of the phenotype is greatly facilitated through pedagogy and other means of culturally entraining the individual to understand and utilize social cooperation at this level and of policing and punishing cheating. We are not natural reciprocators, cooperators, traders, or dividers of our labor. We must learn to do these things, and even despite learning, some ongoing mechanism for policing and punishing cheating seems necessary. But we learn and adopt them because of a mind prepared to do so by its possession of the instrumental capacities for EF. EF provides a means to understand the rational basis for human cooperation and to foresee its benefits. Individuals without EF or with greatly impaired or underdeveloped EF simply are incapable of training up to this level of the extended phenotype.

When it is no longer in someone's self-interest to engage in division of labor and trade with particular others, he or she will not continue to do so. The fabric of the particular cooperative will wither and dissolve (Brown & Vincent, 2008). The individuals will go their separate ways or seek out new cooperative ventures and communities or create new forms of government that provide for these preconditions and the principles of voluntary cooperation with division of labor and trade.

Such an analysis makes it evident that people do not pursue a group-living, cooperative, existence because of some innate need to bond or cooperate with others. Cooperative action is situational and group specific. Nor do they do so because of some spiritual quest for oneness of humanity or because of some utopian vision to perfect humankind. They do so *voluntarily* out of purely rational self-interest *when extended over a long view of their life.* They have foresight and so can realize that each is far better off and can achieve more goals more efficiently (Brown & Vincent, 2008) and more likely by engaging in a division of labor with trade (Mises, 1990; Ridley, Matt, 2010). So they are far better off cooperating peaceably with others than by trying to be entirely self-reliant, struggling with each other, or by competing and warring with others over an inequality of resources. The capacity for contemplating long-term self-interest by itself readily explains the cultural evolution of cooperation, division of labor, and more permanent communities, without any need to invoke innate drives, spiritual quests, a benevolent king, or a supernatural supervising entity. When it is no longer in enough individuals' long-term self-interests to cooperate, then cooperation among those people dissolves.

The extended phenotype of EF is dynamic, not static. New levels can arise and disintegrate as a function of the social scaffolding needed to attain and retain it and the fulfillment of individuals' rational self-interests. Certainly damage to the PFC may undermine an individual's ability to participate at this societal level of the extended phenotype. But just as often damage to the cultural-social scaffolding can result in the inability of entire groups of individuals to participate at this level.

Far less is known or appreciated about this level of EF within the field of neuropsychology, but it exists nonetheless in the related fields of social psychology, ethics, business, politics, and economics with which neuropsychology must someday be integrated (Symons, 1992; Tooby & Cosmides, 1992). This level is evident in the obvious practice of individuals engaging in self-improvement, education, financial management, time management, and health maintenance, as these are carried out in groups of self-interested cooperators.

A Second Possible Stage to the
Strategic–Cooperative Level: Principled–Mutualistic

Within the Strategic–Cooperative level of EF may develop a second stage of even higher-level functioning in some individuals and societies. Functioning at this level requires the most far-reaching degrees of foresight (the time horizon) of which humans are capable. It includes the recognition and contemplation of one's own mortality to such a degree that various subsets of complex activities are being undertaken, as in gaining insurance, retirement planning and saving, long-term health maintenance, preventive medicine, corrective medical regimes, and estate planning. No other species engages in the intentional contemplation of transferring the wealth accumulated over a lifetime to offspring. This degree of forethought is accompanied by the longest-term goals humans are capable of imagining, with the greatest capacity for deferred gratification humans can muster. The entire sweep of a human life, of subsequent generations, and even the history of humanity become relevant to one's considerations.

   The level of abstractness of the rules considered, adopted, and implemented here reach the highest levels of which humans are capable— those of essential and universal ethics, macroeconomics, philosophies, constitutions and forms of government, to name a few. The founding documents used to create an entire town, state, or country's government arise from this level of the human extended phenotype of EF/SR.

   Consider the massive complexity of hierarchically organized and nested sets of behavior needed to adhere to highly abstract rules. These rules include, for example, codes of ethics and professional conduct, practice guidelines and standards of care for professions, religious and professional codes of ethics, legal statutes, and even higher-order principles such as those set forth in a government's Bill of Rights that constrain people in government from interfering in the affairs of individuals, such as freedom of the press and of religion, freedom of association, and freedom from illegal search and seizure. Here, sets of strategies are being combined to form higher-order principles of human conduct in our extended chain of action that began at methods, progressed to tactics, moved on to strategies, and now form principles.

Those principles are applied to far larger social groups than the term "cooperative" can readily convey. Communities, townships, cities, states, and countries or unions of countries may form around such abstract principles as a consequence of this level of human EF activity and the span of time and distance over which the future is being contemplated and pursued. All this implies that the fullest or most complete level of human brain maturation is likely not attained until the third to fourth decade of human life.

The degree of cultural scaffolding increases with each move up the phenotypic hierarchy. Some human groups, communities, or societies may not be able to attain or sustain this level of the EF extended phenotype because they have been unable, for whatever reason, to make use of cultural scaffolding (inherited knowledge and inventions). Culture is essential at this level because it provides the overarching principles for mutual self-organization among individuals who are pursuing their long-term welfare. For example, to pursue shorter-term goals one needs methods and follows rules, as in a recipe. Either the individual discovers them, or the surrounding culture provides instruction in them. For mid-term self-interests, particularly that involving others, one needs tactics (sets of methods or rules) that again can be self-discovered or adopted via cultural training. For longer-term self-interests, one needs strategies; these take time to discover and so are far more likely to arise out of a cultural history of prior generations than to be discovered anew in an individual's short lifetime. For the longest-term self-interests, the depth of prior experience needed to develop the principles will almost of necessity require the experience of generations. Higher-order principles being followed at this level of the EF phenotype require generations of trials of various forms of social organization to discover those that are most likely to contribute to an individual's welfare and happiness over the long term of human lives.

The level of social or group complexity operating at this level is not just larger; its very nature is in one sense quite distinctive. It is characterized not only by *extended periods* of cooperative ventures across multiple mutual goals and multiple cooperative groups. It is when people take into consideration the welfare of others and *voluntarily* place it on an equal if not a higher footing with their own self-interests and welfare. Up until now it has been every person pursuing his or her own long-term self-interests even at the level of cooperative groups. But here there is a change in priorities. It represents the concept of *mutualism*.

This stage of the Strategic–Cooperative level of the EF phenotype can now be extended further outward as follow:

CNS pre-executive functions → CNS executive (self-regulatory) functions → executive (self-regulatory) adaptive behavior → self-organization of environmental arrangements (methods, products, artifacts) → self-organizing reciprocal exchanges with others → arranging cooperative ventures with others (and division of labor with trade) → mutualistic living with others

Social Mutualism

Often included with discussions of social cooperation, the term "mutualism" refers to a more abstract principle that is recognized only when very long spans of time are contemplated and only after much experience in the organization of social groups and their interactions has been attained. In cooperative ventures, individuals pursue their own self-interests collectively in a group of like-minded self-interested participants, as in pursuing some common goal and often using division of labor. There is a midterm or later payoff for each for engaging in the cooperative venture toward a common goal. It arises out of no other motive than self-interest, albeit over a much longer term than self-reliance or reciprocity. Mutualism, like cooperative formation, involves like-minded self-interested individuals joining together in pursuit of a common goal. But it differs in that individuals voluntarily place the self-interests of the other member(s) of the venture *equal to or ahead of their own*. This requires initially subordinating or sacrificing immediate or even midterm self-interests to those of the other participants. In doing so, the individual has more to gain over the longer term than was the case in lower-level cooperative or reciprocal social interactions. Granted it is all being done in the long run for one's longer-term self-interests as they perceive that to be. But it is a strategy that places the interests of others on an even higher footing of personal concern than did prior levels. Mutualism can only work when each of the group members behaves in a similarly mutualistic way; otherwise it will break down from any cheaters or free-riders.

Mutualism is a symbiotic activity in which each party, by contributing to the longer-term self-interests of others, gains longer-term advantages for themselves as well. As Hazlitt (1998) trenchantly argued, mutualism may be an effective long-term strategy for maintaining peaceful, moral, and reasonably well-functioning social groups. All members of the group have come to understand that over the long term the self-interests of any individual nearly always converge with the long-term self-interests of others. Hence by looking out for the interests of others in the nearer term, all are likely to reap a greater but longer-term benefit to their own welfare. From such considerations occasional acts of altruistic behavior (one-sided self-sacrifice) may spring and be explained as the consideration of long-term mutual self-interest. Such mutualistic behavior, as many philosophers have argued, is the foundation of the highest level of human ethics and morality, as well as of economics and governments.

The discovery and implementation of such a principle requires all of the preconditions necessary for cooperation, plus an additional one: a shift in the prioritization of goals. It involves the capacity to act in opposition to your own short- *and* midterm self-interests for the sake of the longer-term self-interests of yourself and *another person or persons.* It is the type of behavior often seen in close military units, especially in battle, and in some people in a town, city, state, or even nation when under attack from outsiders or during extensive natural disasters that have affected the region. The individual comes to understand that in the longest run, across decades and even lifetimes, all individuals will fare better in their own longest-term self-interests if they all act with the *long-term* best interests of others in mind. The payoff for doing so is a higher level of both peace and prosperity than in just a shorter-term cooperative group that does not follow this principle. Like-minded people who appreciate the benefits of such a voluntary social policy will seek out other like-minded individuals forming voluntary communities of association in which all practice the principle of looking out for the mutual long-term self-interests of each other.

Social mutualism as practiced in large human groups creates communities of individuals who not only engage in acts from which are derived mutual long-term self-interests and goals. They formulate new levels of rules, organizations, and even governments that permit and support such mutual interests. At this level, laws, rights, community resources and obligations, political parties and special interest groups, economic monetary systems, and other complex social institutions and resources may develop. They will require individuals to take the longest-term view possible for them to contemplate which may in fact span decades to a lifetime.

This is not to say that within such societies smaller cooperatives may not exist that fail to play by this same principle and that even attempt to game the system for their own advantage. For instance, special interest groups may lobby governments for special considerations that place others in the society at a disadvantage. Individuals or groups may file false billing statements to the federal government for medical claims within a government-funded health care system, and businesses may overbill or fraudulently bill or otherwise obtain funds from the public treasury for their own narrow self-interests. The examples here of cheating or free-riding on a system of mutualism are countless and illustrate just how unstable or short lived such a system, if poorly designed, may be. Thus the practice of mutualism may be unattainable or unsustainable at federal or even state levels. But at the level of smaller groups or even communities in which policing of individual behavior against cheaters and corresponding detection and punishment can be more easily implemented, in which apparent similarities can be heightened and dissimilarities reduced, in which shared self-interest is more evident to all, and in which the benefits to all can be more fairly accorded, mutualism may have a chance to blossom. Indeed, given that this is the highest level of cooperative activity requiring high levels of EF and of a culture to support it, this level of functioning would be especially sporadic, unstable, and highly prone to invasion from within or without by people acting at lower levels of the EF hierarchy and for their own nearer-term self-interests. In that sense, it is more of an ideal that individuals and smaller groups may strive for than one that can be stabilized and sustained in practice across generations at the level of far larger groups, cities, states, or even countries. This may be evident in the history of failed settlements, colonies, cities, states, countries, and even collapses of entire civilizations.

Does Religion Have a Role in the Origins of Social Cooperatives and Mutualism?

It has recently been argued (McCullough & Carter, 2011; McCullough & Willoughby, 2009) that religions may have evolved in human cultural history to facilitate self-regulation at this level of the EF phenotype in community activities. Religious doctrines, moral codes, and the belief in a supernatural agent who monitors conduct and eventually dispenses consequences may have facilitated more peaceful within-group coexistence at the level of communities (Rossano, 2007). Religions appear to emphasize delay of gratification, tolerance of others, and social cooperation within the group. Such religious principles may operate to boost individual EF/SR as it is practiced among large groups of individuals dwelling in close proximity. Religions also emphasize mutual monitoring of one's behavior by others and by a hypothetical supernatural deity, both of which may contribute to self-regulation or at least its motivational basis. It is an interesting hypothesis worthy of further exploration.

The religious doctrines that promote within-group cooperation and harmony can exacerbate between-group enmity and aggression. Recall that some of the preconditions for voluntary cooperation to arise are shared self-interests (and the perception of such in humans), a heightening of one's similarities to others (shared self-interests), and a diminution of individual differences (unshared self-interests). A religion may provide these conditions within a community that has adopted that religion, but dissimilarities are heightened when groups having different religions come into contact with each other. Religion is then no longer a force for cooperation but for aggression. For opposing religious communities to eventually cooperate, their dissimilarities would need to be minimized and the similarities maximized. Currently humanity appears to be experimenting with various means to minimize conflicts among religions; however, the growing human population and greater flow of information and trade make group contacts and conflicts among religions inevitable.

Apart from its potential role in facilitating within-group cooperation, religion may facilitate or boost the likely success of EF/SR. It may do so through its encouragement of deferred gratification and through its belief that a supernatural agent is monitoring the person's actions (Shermer, 2011).

Conclusions

EF is self-regulation across time to direct and sustain goal-directed action in the context of others, often relying on social means. Yet given what has transpired to produce this higher level of the EF phenotype, we can now amend the definition yet again: *the use of self-directed actions so as to choose goals and to select, enact, and sustain actions across time toward those goals usually in the context of others, often relying on social **and cultural means.***

This level of EF is illustrated in Figure 7.1, which shows the natural progression to this level. The level can be identified by the increases needed in the eight developmental parameters that characterized lower levels. The level of neurological maturation needed to function at this level is quite advanced and probably dependent on full brain maturation.

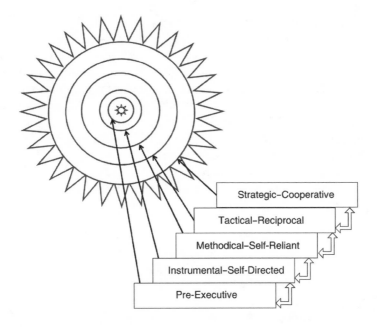

FIGURE 7.1. Two different ways of illustrating the extended EF phenotype as it occurs at the Strategic–Cooperative level. The concentric rings at the left indicate the outwardly radiating nature of the phenotype at this fifth stage of development (Pre-Executive, Instrumental–Self-Directed, Methodical–Self-Reliant, Tactical–Reciprocal, Strategic–Cooperative). The stacked boxes at the lower right indicate the hierarchical arrangement of these five phenotypic levels. Information from the lower levels flows upward to the higher levels while management of the lower levels may be exerted downward by the next higher level.

The extent to which the physical and social environments are being rearranged is far greater than lower levels, more fluid, and more protracted. It may even include the formal physical codification of conditions, rules, or terms, and consequences as in contracts and laws that serve to facilitate this level of EF/SR among members of the group (i.e., culture). The *spatial* and *temporal* horizons needed here are more extensive than is evident at lower levels. The time horizon of foresight, for example, may involve months and even years. The extent to which delayed consequences are valued must also increase in salience to *motivate* highly complex, extended chains of behavior over lengthy periods of time. The level of general, *abstract* rules that are developed and followed is greater than at any prior level of the EF phenotype. The degree of *behavioral* complexity that is needed here is also very high—and certainly more complex than that evident at lower levels. Clearly the need for and complexity of interactions with the *social* group at this level of EF is likewise considerable. All this is facilitated by *cultural* scaffolding from previous generations and the creation of new cultural means. This may lead to a final stage within this level under some conditions in small groups, the Principled–Mutualistic level of the extended EF phenotype model—one not attained by all individuals or even social groups. It is a level at which an individual places the self-interests of others on an equal or higher priority than his or her own and thus all voluntarily act with each other's longer-term self-interests in mind.

8

The Extended Utilitarian Zone

The effects of the full extended phenotype of EF continue to radiate outward. This zone of radiating effects contains long-term consequences for EF/SR in an individual. It essentially asks the questions: Did using EF/SR work? If so, how well? Looking at EF as an evolutionary adaptation across our species, the answer to the first question has to be yes. If EF/SR had failed to achieve any benefit for the individual, it would not have become a stable trait in the human genotype or phenotype. At each new level of EF, consequences (advantages mostly) accrue to the individual; otherwise, the extension into that zone of effects would either not have happened or it would be a mere by-product with no effect, and therefore it would not be considered part of the extended EF phenotype at all. Recall from Chapter 2 that by-products must have effects that alter survival, reproduction, inclusive fitness, or self-interests generally, or they are not considered extended phenotypic effects. Therefore, each new ring of the phenotype is surrounded by a feedback zone of adaptive effects.

In short, extended phenotypes produce extended consequences. I refer to this outermost zone of consequences as the Extended Utilitarian zone. These consequences are part of the phenotype because they are the feedback mechanism—the consequences for human survival and welfare for using EF/SR.

More proximal consequences, of course, arose at each level of the extended EF phenotype described previously. Here, I wish to concentrate on the longer or longest term, furthest reaching effects-at-a-distance for using EF/SR at all prior levels and zones over extended periods of time. After decades of using EF/SR to pursue goals, how well or poorly has the individual succeeded? Has using EF/SR or not paid off in the long run? The final arbiter of that judgment can only be the person, because it is a question of subjective use-value as described in Chapter 4. However, there are some objective measures that can be used by others to answer this question. The following suggests a number of ways to gather objective data for answering these questions.

Objective Means of Judging
Extended EF Phenotypic Effects

Effects on Survival

If one evolutionary purpose of the EF/SR system is improved survival, then we can objectively ask how well it has worked to sustain a human's life. Advances in culture (hygiene, living conditions, public health, medicine, psychology, etc.) have clearly contributed to improvements in average human life expectancies in developed countries across the centuries. Those cultural advances were created by the use of the EF/SR system (reason and science). Improvements in average life expectancy provide potential metrics for evaluating the utility of EF/SR objectively.

Increased knowledge about sources of health and illness allow members of the culture to make lifestyle choices using their EF/SR system. Smoking, drinking alcohol, drug abuse, criminal behavior, lack of exercise, excessive eating that leads to obesity or diabetes, reckless driving, and risk-taking generally are all publicly observable forms of behavior that have adverse consequences. All of them have been shown to be in part related to one's degree of using EF/SR as rated in daily life (Barkley, 2011a). All of them in varying degrees impact health and life expectancy, often through higher risks for accidents, cardiovascular disease, and cancer. Therefore, the degree to which these may have directly contributed to shortened life expectancy and the extent to which EF/SR or its deficiency led to these behavior patterns and impairments can be considered metrics for how well EF/SR works to promote long-term welfare.

Let us first consider life expectancy. EF is directly related to that dimension of personality known as conscientiousness—an aspect of personality reflecting how likely one is to consider the consequences of one's actions for self and others before acting. Its opposite is impulsiveness and selfishness. Lower levels of conscientiousness have been linked repeatedly to health problems and even to life expectancy (Friedman et al., 1995). Swensen and colleagues (2004) have found that adults with ADHD who have substantial deficits in EF (Barkley & Murphy, 2010) are more than twice as likely to die prematurely from misadventures compared to control cases. Children with high impulsivity, among other problem behaviors, were also more likely to die by 46 years of age than were children low in these attributes. The risk for children in the highest quartile of impulsiveness and related externalizing behavior (3.2%) was more than double that of children in the lowest quartile (1.4%) (Jokela, Ferrie, & Kivimaki, 2009).

Friedman and colleagues (Friedman et al., 1995) followed up Terman's original sample of highly intelligent children across their lifespans. That study also demonstrated the link between low childhood conscientiousness (low EF; high impulsivity) and shortened life expectancy. More than half of the sample was deceased at the time of follow-up (pre–1995), with most of the surviving participants in their 80s or older. The follow-up study indicated that the most significant childhood personality characteristic predictive of reduced life expectancy by all causes was related to the impulsive, undercontrolled personality characteristics of low conscientiousness. Individuals classified as falling in this lowest quartile of conscientiousness (being highly impulsive) on this set of characteristics lived an average of 8 years less than those who did not (73 vs. 81 years). Deaths among the study participants were most often due to cardiovascular disease or cancer, the two most common killers in the United States today. Friedman et al. (1995) provided data to show that low childhood conscientiousness is linked to these diseases through its impact on lifestyle choices, such as smoking, drinking, exercise, weight, and cholesterol management. That conclusion would seem to be further supported by the fact that Terman's participants were also intellectually gifted and came from families of above-average or higher economic backgrounds. Both of these factors probably would have conveyed a greater advantage toward longer life expectancy than would be the case for intellectually normal children or adults. Thus, there is some reason to suspect that health, lifestyle, and life expectancy may be adversely affected as a function of deficits in EF/SR.

This inference was directly demonstrated recently in three separate studies of the relationship of ratings of EF/SR deficits in daily life and impairment in numerous domains of major life activities (Barkley, 2011a; Barkley & Fischer, 2011; Barkley & Murphy, 2010, 2011). The first study examined EF deficits in adults with ADHD and in clinical and community control adults. A second study followed children with ADHD and control children to young adulthood, and the third study focused on a general population sample of 1,240 adults ages 18–81 in the United States. These studies showed significant relationships between ratings of EF deficits and the following domains: employment status and occupational functioning; educational attainment, academic performance, and school functioning; household income; marital status and satisfaction; parenting stress; offspring psychiatric morbidity; driving risks; financial problems and credit rating; criminal behavior and arrest rates; health concerns; psychopathology; and general ratings of impairment in life activities across 15 domains of functioning. The extended phenotypic effects of EF and its deficits clearly project well beyond the skin and brain functioning to impart adverse effects in many major life activities and at distances from the genotype highly consistent with the extended phenotype concept and its application here to understanding EF.

Others' Recollections and Judgments: Consequences at a Distance

It is reasonable to propose that the extent to which an individual possesses and utilizes EF can also be indexed by two other sources and that these reflect extended phenotypic effects. The first source is the memory of others with whom a person has repeatedly interacted. The recollections of others and their judgments about an individual's use of EF/SR in daily life are legitimate sources for detecting the effects of EF at a distance, in this case on another's judgments of one's social conduct. Ratings of others about a person on an EF rating scale can serve this purpose. They have been shown to be significantly predictive of results in many of the same domains of major life activities reported above using self-reported ratings of EF deficits (Barkley, 2011a). How can these reports of others be considered phenotypic effects? Such recollections and ratings of others can readily determine whether or not the person being rated will be interacted with, reciprocated with, and cooperated with by those who hold the recollections. Those judgments may also impact the likelihood that the person so evaluated may be promoted in educational settings and graduate with the intended terminal degree, succeed in employment settings, gain access into community organizations, clubs, or other formal social gatherings, retain their licenses to drive and practice their occupational specialty, be granted loans by credit institutions, succeed in their marriages, get custody of or visitation with their children if divorced, and so on. Countless opportunities in life hinge directly on the judgments of others about an individual's degree of EF, even if assessed only indirectly via their social conduct and handling of daily responsibilities. Such social judgments and their attendant consequences have a direct bearing on an individual's survival, reproduction, and long-term welfare. Therefore, to the extent they affect the person's survival and welfare, they are phenotypic effects. In short, the recollections and judgments of others about an individual provide a convincing means of evaluating the extended phenotypic effects of EF on numerous domains of major life activities.

Archival Records and Their Consequences

Another means of evaluating extended phenotypic effects is through the archival records accumulated across an individual's life. These may include health records, school reports and records, driving records, criminal records, military service records, employment status and records, insurance and workman's compensation claims, credit reports, civil court proceedings, and other archives that reflect "the paper trail" of an individual's life and the consequences they experience. Many of those consequences directly or indirectly reflect the extent to which the individual possesses and uses EF at the various levels of the extended phenotype. As previously explicated, EF can be extended upward and outward from an individual through their self-reliant, reciprocal, cooperative, and mutualistic behavior in domains of life activity. All of these levels and associated activities are connected through foresight—the person's capacity to contemplate the long-term consequences of actions for self and others and act accordingly.

As already discussed, archived records showing impaired functioning of an individual in daily life and the negative consequences for that person are significantly associated with the person's degree of EF deficits, whether self-reported or rated by others who know him or her well (Barkley, 2011a). It is not farfetched to suggest that the archival records associated with an individual's life are part of the extended EF phenotype. They are, after all, effects of that phenotype to varying degrees because they have consequences that can feed back to the individual's long-term welfare for good or ill. Those consequences make records part of the extended EF phenotype.

These records have consequences for an individual seeking to further participate in any of the domains of major life activities. One cannot get into college or the military without a high school diploma or graduate equivalency degree and the transcript that supports it. A criminal record, a bad credit score, a terrible driving record—each has adverse effects for the person's future welfare. In this way they not only reflect the extended phenotypic effects of prior EF but can also be such effects going forward.

Effects of EF on Offspring Survival and Welfare

One extended phenotypic effect that may exist in humans, as well as in other species, is the impact on survival, reproduction, and long-term welfare of offspring. While this is often considered under the concept of inclusive fitness (the welfare of the shared genetics among relatives), here I wish to consider the environmental impact of an individual's EF phenotype on the resources and survival opportunities for offspring. An individual's capacity for EF/SR has an effect on the degree of distress he or she reports in the role of parent. It is not hard to imagine that there is also a direct impact on their parenting behavior specifically. This might then affect offspring survival and general welfare. Parents low in EF and the related trait of conscientiousness may provide less safe, less enriching, and otherwise less nurturing and supportive environments that interfere with growth, development, general welfare, and even survival of the offspring apart from any shared genetics that exist between the two parties. Although EF has not been well studied in its relationship to parenting behavior, offspring adjustment, and general offspring welfare, it is not difficult to conceive of the adverse effects EF deficits would have on this important role in adult life.

There is indirect evidence for such an effect. As noted above, ADHD is associated with substantial deficits in virtually all components of EF as rated in daily life activities (Barkley, 2011a)—so much so that some investigators (myself included) now consider the disorder to be one of EF (Barkley, 1997a, 1997b; Barkley & Murphy, 2010; Brown, 2006; Wolf & Wasserstein, 2001). Consequently, findings pertinent to parenting by adults with ADHD could be linked to their EF deficits that comprise their ADHD symptoms. Parents with ADHD may have a greater difficulty coping with children and family life more generally than do those without ADHD, as suggested above. Studies by Eric Mash and his students have shed further light on this issue, suggesting that these differences may even be evident among women who are expecting their first child. Ninowski, Mash, and Benzies (2007) reported a comparison of expectant mothers who reported high levels of ADHD symptoms compared to those with lower levels. They found that women with high ADHD severity were less likely to be married, less likely to have gone to college, and less likely to report that they wanted to get pregnant. Level of ADHD symptoms was associated with greater anxiety and depression and less positive expectations about their soon-to-be-born infant and their future maternal role. My colleagues and I also found adult women with ADHD to be less likely to be married (Barkley et al., 2008).

Watson and Mash (in press) continued this line of research by evaluating women with young infants for their level of ADHD symptoms and its association with maternal–child relations. Again, they found that ADHD severity was associated with higher levels of anxiety and depression, and also contributed to higher levels of maternal hostile–reactive behavior in mothers who had difficult infants. The level of maternal ADHD had no effect on perceived parental self-efficacy after controlling for parental anxiety and depression. But maternal ADHD severity was associated with a reduced sense of perceived parental impact on child behavior. Perceived social support was unrelated to maternal ADHD symptoms.

The effect of maternal ADHD symptoms was further examined in a study by Banks, Ninowski, Mash, and Semple (2008) who compared women high in levels of ADHD symptoms with those with lower levels. Women high in ADHD symptoms had more occupational and psychiatric problems, lower parenting self-esteem, and a more external locus of control for their parenting. They also reported less effective disciplinary styles than did women low in ADHD symptoms. While none of these studies used clinically referred women diagnosed with ADHD, they clearly suggest that ADHD in women is likely to have an adverse impact on their parenting, on parental stress, and on parent–child interactions.

Further adverse effects of adult ADHD on parental roles and functioning were found by Murray and Johnston (2006) who compared mothers with and without ADHD who all had children with ADHD on various parenting measures and parent–child interaction measures. The mothers with ADHD appeared to be less effective at problem solving around child behavior issues than control mothers. Results remained the same even after controlling for severity of child oppositional defiant disorder and conduct disorder symptoms. The mothers with ADHD were also found to be poorer at monitoring child behavior and less consistent disciplinarians relative to mothers without the disorder. Poor parental monitoring of child behavior is a risk factor for accidental injuries and may help to explain the elevated rates of such injuries in children with ADHD (Barkley, 2006), given that parental ADHD may be one source for such lowered levels of child monitoring. Similar adverse effects of maternal ADHD on parenting were also reported by Chronis-Toscano and colleagues (2008). Given that 85–96% of adults with ADHD are impaired (below the 7th percentile) in one or more domains of EF as rated in daily life activities, then these findings have a direct bearing on the likelihood that the degree and quality of EF have effects on parenting behavior and hence on offspring risk and welfare. This would represent yet another extended EF phenotypic effect at this Extended Utilitarian level.

Apart from such direct effects of parental EF/SR on offspring survival and welfare, there are indirect effects that most likely occur as a function of the extended EF phenotype. Humans are one of the few species that not only transfer learning to their offspring via pedagogy during parents' lifetime, they also make their resources available to offspring during their lifetime and even transfer such assets to their offspring upon their own demise. In view of the effects of EF on occupational functioning, education, socioeconomic status, and income among other domains of life discussed above, it is not difficult to see that individuals higher or lower in EF/SR would have greater or lesser resources to make available to their offspring at these stages of life. It is difficult to imagine that parental resources transferred to offspring do not have some effects on the likelihood of offspring survival. Nevertheless, they certainly contribute to health and welfare in offspring and may even contribute to the likelihood that those offspring will mate, the qualities those mates will possess, their own reproduction, and whether they continue the genetic line. All this is to say that the extended EF phenotype can have both direct and indirect effects on offspring viability, survival, welfare, and their own eventual reproductive success. All of these effects feed back onto the parent EF genotype.

Conclusions

The adaptive success of the degree of EF displayed by individuals can be evaluated in the recollections and judgments of others as well as in the archival records that reflect personal achievements and failures, wealth and poverty, health and lifespan. EF impairments are likely to be experienced in major life domains over a lifetime.

Societies and cultural institutions can also be judged for the extent to which their policies and practices promote, retard, preclude, or snuff out the adaptive effects of the extended EF phenotype. How successful or effective is the cultural scaffolding available to the individual for the promotion of these extended phenotypic actions and effects? One can then judge how well these effects promote human survival, long-term happiness, and welfare. The further outward one progresses in extended phenotypic zones, the more culture must provide the scaffolding to reach the next zone of actions and effects. Some types of cultural scaffolding may be better than others at promoting human EF, self-regulation, self-determination, and the individual's success at pursuing their long-term happiness and welfare. Some rules and policies, cultural practices, devices, products, and knowledge promote extended EF actions while others distort, pervert, retard, or regress them. To the extent that states or societies promote the rights of individuals to pursue their long-term welfare as they determine it to be, then those institutions will be consilient with the promotion of the extended EF phenotype.

The standard for judging them is the final definition of EF worth reiterating: *the use of self-directed actions so as to choose goals and to select, enact, and sustain actions across time toward those goals usually in the context of others often relying on social and cultural means for the maximization of one's long-term welfare as the person defines that to be.*

Figure 8.1 illustrates this final level of the extended EF phenotype. The sunburst perimeter around the concentric rings on the left is intended to convey this final zone of radiating influence of EF as used across long

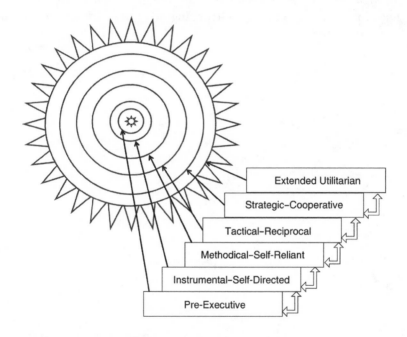

FIGURE 8.1. Two different ways of illustrating the extended EF phenotype as it occurs at the Extended Utilitarian level. The concentric rings at the left indicate the outwardly radiating nature of the phenotype at this final stage of development (Pre-Executive, Instrumental–Self-Directed, Methodical–Self-Reliant, Tactical–Reciprocal, Strategic–Cooperative, Principled–Mutualistic), as does the leftward-pointing arrow. The final sunburst edging of this diagram reflects the extended consequences or utility of employing EF across these levels and one's lifetime. The stacked boxes at the right indicate the hierarchical arrangement of these six phenotypic levels and the ultimate utility (effects-at-a-distance) of using them. The bidirectional arrows to the right of each box are intended to convey the bidirectional flow of information between the levels. Information from the lower levels flows upward to the higher levels, while management of the lower levels may be exerted downward by the next higher level.

intervals of one's life. The diagram on the right once again reflects the stepwise increments in the EF phenotypic hierarchy. By adulthood, EF is mature along with its developmental capacities, and all rings of the extended EF phenotype are present. This model should be considered as a totality in evaluating EF in adult life. Adults pursue various goals, at varying distances across time and space, using various social means such as reciprocity, exchange, trade, cooperation, and mutualism as well as various cultural means (rules, laws, ethical principles, etc.) and products or inventions. Therefore phenotypic effects can be seen across all of the zones in a mature normally functioning adult with EF depending on these parameters.

9

Implications for Understanding Executive Functioning and Its Disorders

This book was written to address four related problems that currently exist in the concept of EF, as initially presented in Chapter 1. This chapter and the next consider whether those problems have been addressed. The issues of a definition of EF, of inadequate theories, and of the purpose of EF are covered here. How to assess EF is discussed in the next chapter, as are the implications of this theory for the management of disorders of EF.

The Problem of Defining EF

The first problem was the lack of an explicit operational definition of EF. Which human mental functions can be considered executive in nature and which ones cannot? In short, "What is EF?" I began by using the statement that EF is self-regulation (EF = SR), given the general consensus in the field of neuropsychology on the matter. Other definitions, such as that by Welsh and Pennington (1988) that actually derived from Luria (1966) and through him back to Bekhterev (1905), were viewed as inadequate as an operational definition. That is because they employed terms so ambiguous (i.e., "the ability," "appropriate," "those processes," etc.) as to be unable to be used as criteria to determine what components, functions, or processes are or are not "executive" in nature. Some also limited the definition of EF to simply that of sustaining problem solving toward goals. Problem solving is only one type or component of EF according to various earlier models and not its sole or essential nature. The origin of these processes in the PFC as a basis for defining EF is a nonstarter.

The present model of EF solves this problem by first of all substituting the more specific definition of self-regulation as that of EF: directing an action to the self that modifies a subsequent action or behavior so as to alter a delayed consequence (attain a goal). There are several forms or components of EF because people can direct several actions back at themselves so as to regulate their own behavior toward their goals. I then specified that each component of EF (types of self-regulation) arise out of two developmental processes: the *self-direction of actions* and their *internalization*. It is the self-direction of human actions that makes an act, function, or component executive in nature. Self-directed action is done to alter subsequent behavior from what it would have otherwise been—it is a means to an end. It is done to alter the likelihood of future consequences for the individual (to attain various ends or goals). This constitutes the basic or starting definition of self-regulation. Therefore, the initial definition of EF was clarified and made more specific as follows: *EF is the use of self-directed actions so as to choose goals and to select, enact, and sustain actions across time toward those goals* (Chapter 3). Although the cross-temporal nature of EF is implied in the definition of self-regulation, it was important to make it explicit. Humans bind current status, intermediate means, and future ends together into cross-temporal structures that are mentally represented and serve to guide goal-directed actions (Fuster, 1997).

Six self-directed actions were identified as used by humans for self-regulation. They are the components of EF: Self-directed attention to create self-awareness, self-directed inhibition to create self-restraint, self-directed sensory–motor actions to create mental representations and simulations (ideation), self-directed speech to create verbal thinking, self-directed emotion and motivation to create conscious appraisal, and self-directed play (nonverbal and verbal reconstitution) to create problem solving, fluency, or innovation. Humans use at least six forms of self-regulation in directing and sustaining action toward a goal. Each is an EF as defined here. The term "EF" as used here therefore includes the concept of problem solving as it occurs in the Welsh and Pennington definition above but is more inclusive in bringing into the construct of EF the other components as well. Those authors and others tried to do much the same by subsequently specifying that EF included working memory and inhibition as its principal components. While I agree, I pre-

fer to redefine each as self-directed actions to make it clear why they are
EF in nature and why other brain activities or functions are not (they are
not self-directed to modify behavior to attain goals and to choose, enact,
and sustain the means needed to reach those goals). Moreover, these
authors failed to note the critical role of both self-awareness and self-
appraisal (self-directed emotion and motivation) in EF as self-regulation;
they are the mechanisms by which the individual even possesses a sense
of self that requires modification as well as for the rapid cost-benefit calculations with regard to various ends and means being contemplated by
and for the self, respectively.

Using the extended phenotype viewpoint, EF was examined for
its radiating effects outside of the individual at spatial and temporal
distances into the person's natural ecology. This led to an appreciation
for the important role of EF at the Methodical–Self-Reliant level of
the EF phenotype. This level and its zone of effects respects the group-
living niche in which humans exist and so includes other humans as
self-interested competitors and manipulators that occupy that niche
and so create problems and opportunities for the individual. Fellow
humans are likely to be engaging in the parasitic manipulation of others as tools (means) to attain goals (ends). Thus, the definition of EF
was broadened to incorporate this initial social context, and became
*the use of self-directed actions so as to choose goals and to select,
enact, and sustain actions across time toward those goals usually in
the context of others.*

As the subsequent radiating zones or levels of the extended EF phenotype were identified, it became evident that EF is not just indispens-
able for social predation and self-defense and so for independence from
others (self-reliance). By taking a longer view of one's self-interests, one
could conceive of using others as a means to goals in a symbiotic manner
that was more beneficial to both parties than being self-reliant or parasitic. This connected EF to the universal human practice of reciprocity
and exchange, (the Tactical–Reciprocal level). By further extending the
time horizon over which one contemplates goals, it is possible to show
that reciprocity could be improved through forming cooperatives (social
groups that act as a single interdependent unit, such as in unison, to
accomplish shared goals). From there I showed how such cooperatives,
if sustained over sufficient time, would eventually result in a division of
labor with trade among its members (the Strategic–Cooperative level).
To gain from this arrangement, each member of the cooperative must
sacrifice some of their own independence and self-reliance so as to specialize in an activity of value to the members and then engage in trading

their surpluses for the products and services of the other specialist members. The group acts as a unity with specialization and exchange among its component parts. Understanding these extended phenotypic effects of EF led to a further expansion of the definition of EF as follows: *the use of self-directed actions so as to choose goals and to select, enact, and sustain actions across time toward those goals usually in the context of others **often relying on social means.***

Along the way, the extended phenotype model of EF describes an increasing use of cultural scaffolding to ratchet up human capacities for goal-directed actions. Humans create and use culture (stored and shared information)—its knowledge, systems, inventions, devices, and products—to significantly improve their EF capacities for attaining larger goals, extending over longer time spans and spatial distances. Thus, the definition of EF was further expanded to recognize this bidirectional relationship of EF to culture: *the use of self-directed actions so as to choose goals and to select, enact, and sustain actions across time toward those goals usually in the context of others often relying on social **and cultural means.***

Finally, in order to contrast forms of cultural scaffolding (principles, policies, and governments) that do and do not promote the human ability for goal-directed action, it became necessary to emphasize that, like all life, human EF is motivated out of self-interest, albeit over the long term. Such self-interest can only be determined by the individual using their reason. At its core, then, human EF is motivated by subjective appraisal of self-interest and is essentially self-determination. Forms of cultural scaffolding that accept and promote these basic features of human nature allow EF to succeed, extend outward to have wider phenotypic effects, and permit human life to thrive and prosper as individuals pursue their long-term self-interests as they determine those interests to be. EF was therefore concluded to be *the use of self-directed actions so as to choose goals and to select, enact, and sustain actions across time toward those goals usually in the context of others often relying on social and cultural means **for the maximization of one's longer-term welfare as the person defines that to be.*** Such a definition fulfills the requirement set forth at the start that such a definition must be explicit enough to serve as an operational criterion for what is and is not EF (the standard of self-directed actions for purposes of self-regulation). Yet any definition must also be inclusive enough to represent human EF as we find it in everyday life—self-interested, yet in the context of others, involving mutually beneficial interactions and ventures, and relying on culture as a means to self-determined ends. It is left to the reader to decide if this final definition of EF is a marked improvement over earlier ones.

The Problem of the Nature of EF: Incomplete Theories

As argued in Chapter 1, theories are not just constructs, but mechanisms; they give us explanations of relationships among constructs. They are time-limited working models of how reality, in this case EF, operates. Theories address the questions of "How does EF work?" or "What does it do?" Without a coherent theory of EF, the number of constructs involved has risen to 33 or more. If our goals are precision of thinking and definition as well as utility of prediction, this situation is patently unacceptable. Prediction requires propositions about how things relate to each other. Listing a set of constructs that are presumed to make up a "metaconstruct" will not suffice without some operational definition as to what makes that list executive in nature and an explanation of mechanisms as to how the constructs being labeled as EF relate to each other. Without such a definition and explanation, there is no theory of EF. In response to this problem, I have adopted the viewpoint of an extended phenotype as used in evolutionary biology (Dawkins, 1982). It provides a potentially useful means of fleshing out a working theory of EF.

The preceding chapters have explicated an evolutionary developmental viewpoint of EF as an extended phenotype. It arises from a maturational course that likely spans three decades that it may take for the PFC (and the EF system that depends upon it) to reach full maturity in the typical human. The model asserts hierarchical levels of the EF phenotype with an expanding set of effects of human action and interaction at each level. The earlier chapters also discussed some of the effects that this extended EF phenotype produces at both spatial and temporal distances from the genotype that gives rise to this EF system. EF is, after all, a human trait that is universal to the species.

The pre-EF level transitions to the Instrumental–Self-Directed level when certain pre-EF neuropsychological functions start to become self-directed for the purpose of self-regulation. From this arises self-awareness, inhibition, nonverbal and verbal working memory, emotional and motivational self-regulation, and planning and problem solving, which are each conceptualized here as actions-to-the-self. These actions-to-the-self may be overt in early development and yet progress to being privatized, covert, or internalized (mental) in form with maturation through the process of internalization. This process gives rise to forms of private behavior (mental activities) in which humans may engage for self-regulation toward goals.

These EF processes are then used at the next phenotypic level of Methodical–Self-Reliant for day-to-day survival, self-care, self-defense, and independence from others. At this level, EF is conceptualized as involving at least five interrelated dimensions of self-regulation as reflected in observations and ratings of daily EF. These are: self-management across time; self-organization and problem solving; self-restraint (inhibition and self-subordination of short-term self-interests); self-motivation; and self-regulation of emotions. At this level, additional cognitive abilities may emerge along with additional social learning, such as theory of mind, social self-defense, and imitation and vicarious learning via the mirror neuronal system of the PFC. It may also be further demarcated by the self-organization (rearrangement) of external environmental props that facilitate and magnify the cognitive capacities for self-regulation and extend them over longer spans of time.

Progressing upward, the succeeding Tactical–Reciprocal level contributes to daily social exchange and reciprocity as part of group living. This level is demarcated by the larger, longer-term social purposes to which EF is being applied and for which it likely evolved for day-to-day social existence and functioning. This is the beginning connection of EF to economic behavior, markets, and social interdependence for mutual benefit.

This phenotypic level eventually gives rise to the next level of EF effects-at-a-distance: the Strategic–Cooperative level. This level is reached when EF tactics and their goals become means and subgoals to larger, longer-term goals and the more complex behavioral structures needed to attain them. This level is also identified by the use of social cooperatives with division of labor and trade among its members. Individuals join together as a cooperative to act as a unit in which each specializes in a task needed by the members while engaging in exchange with other specialists. The formation of cooperatives that act as a unity using division of labor with trade achieves greater shared benefits and common ends than is the case had each member acted alone as a self-reliant, independent entity merely engaging in exchange of surpluses with others. In doing so, the members of a cooperative capitalize on the variability in human abilities and the variation in natural resources, which leads each to pursue activities for which they may be more adept or have greater access while trading the excesses of their labors with others who are doing the same. This EF level and extended phenotypic effects result in the formation of communities of cooperators living in proximity (having lower dispersal rates) so as to facilitate specialization and trade for mutual benefits. The interdependence of the members of the cooperative has as a by-product the origin of settlements, cities, and eventually societies of self-regulating, goal-directed, self-interested yet interdependent cooperative specialists.

In this last level, Strategic–Cooperative, a second stage may emerge among some cooperatives that extend their activities over sufficient lengths of time and develop sufficient cultural scaffolding to achieve it, and that is the Principled–Mutualistic stage. In it, like-minded individuals pursue their mutual longer term self-interests by putting the self-interests of others initially on an equal footing, if not ahead of their own near-term and midterm self-interests. To succeed, all must practice such mutualism, for it is highly prone to invasion by cheaters and free-riders and hence is very unstable over time. It is essentially the practice of my watching out for your long-term self-interests while you are watching out for mine as we pursue our own self-interests together, as a cooperative. Such mutualists have come to recognize that over the longest term, the vast majority of an individual's self-interests converge on those of others. They do this to achieve even greater benefits for all such participating mutualists that none can achieve individually or even acting as a cooperative. It must be practiced voluntarily, sufficiently widespread across the cooperative, with a heightened sense of shared similarity and a reduced sense of unshared dissimilarities, adequately policed, and with the real threat of group punishment or even expulsion to succeed. To arise and succeed, such an advanced stage of EF requires the greatest capacity for foresight, subordination of immediate self-interests (delay of gratification), and the formation of a highly interdependent social cooperative, with a high level of cultural scaffolding (external information, prolonged pedagogy, organizational systems, rules, products, etc.). All of these levels are surrounded by the outermost zone of effects that reflect the extended utility or proximal, intermediate, and life-long consequences of EF functioning at these various levels.

Over development, the EF phenotype expands outward as the individual's time horizon for contemplation extends further into the probable future. This is *the* common thread that binds all levels of this extended phenotype. It is also the thread that binds EF to the fields of ethics and morality, law, economics, culture, politics and government because all of them depend on this mental faculty for their existence. This is not just the capacity to sense and contemplate the probable future that may come to pass if things remain as they are. It is also the capacity to contemplate the possible future, a future that could result from one's own desires if one elects to plan for it and pursue it. This sense of the possible future leads to a growing preference for larger delayed consequences over smaller immediate ones, often referred to in economics as one's time preference (Kelly, 2010; Mises, 1990; Ridley, Matt, 2010) and in behavior analysis as temporal or reward discounting (Green et al., 1994, 1996). It provides a greater motivation to self-organize and self-sustain goal-directed actions toward those larger delayed consequences. The development of this EF hierarchy results in a progression of behavioral complexity from methods to tactics to strategies and, perhaps for some, onward to principles. Methods for self-reliance can be grouped into sets to form tactics for social exchange and reciprocity that can eventually be organized into sets to form strategies for group organizations like cooperatives, with each transition resulting in longer, more hierarchically organized, more complex, and more temporally extended goal-directed activities.

As a result of the developing capacity for taking "the long view," it becomes evident to individuals that they need each other and can choose to rely on each other if each is to gain the benefits that accrue to reciprocators, cooperators, and mutualists. As a result, the social networks necessary to achieve longer-term goals increase and change in complexity and duration. Across all levels there is also an increase in the level of abstractness of the rules being followed for pursuing one's long-term welfare from methods to tactics to strategies on to the use of principles—the most abstract rules governing human life. Finally, across the levels is a growing reliance on culture as well as contribution to it—the accumulated and shared knowledge, means, methods, systems, devices, and products on which individuals will capitalize to achieve their longer-term goals and to which they will contribute using EF. There is not just utility but grandeur in this view of EF as an extended phenotype.

Numerous theoretical and clinical implications flow from adopting the extended phenotype model of EF/SR and the notion that it has effects-at-a-distance into the social ecology. Many of these implications have been discussed in earlier chapters in explicating each level of the model and so are not reiterated here. But some are worth highlighting to show the distinctive features of this model from previous alternative views of EF. For example, from this theory, one can identify six distinctive properties of the human mind and EF:

1. Prolongation (prolonging sensory representations to form mental images and icons).
2. Separation (decoupling the stimulus from the response via inhibition of the response, thereby inserting a delay in which the event can be further appraised and alternative actions contemplated).
3. Self-direction (six pre-executive abilities have come to be turned back on the individual to produce self-awareness, self-restraint, self-sensory–motor actions, self-speech, self-regulation of emotion and motivation, and self-play for innovation and problem solving).
4. Internalization (the self-directed activities are eventually privatized from public view to form cognitive or mental actions).
5. Symbolization (mental representations became associated with verbal utterances that create symbols that represent aspects of those representations, such as objects, actions, and their properties).
6. Reconstitution (using mental representations, and especially the symbols for them, the environment and one's actions toward it can be classified, categorized, and otherwise taken apart and recombined to form new representations and actions).

One problem with current theories of EF is that they have grown increasingly disparate from descriptions of patients suffering PFC/EF system injuries. Patients with EF deficits (PFC disorders or injuries) have problems with morality, selfishness, rationality, reciprocity, cooperation, mutualism, and social skills, not to mention problems with occupational functioning, economic self-support, managing money, repaying debts, long-term cohabiting relationships, child-rearing, criminal conduct, psychopathic propensities, and even self-reliance (daily adaptive functioning). How do you account for such problems from EF models built on doing digit span backwards or N-back tasks, generating multiple words to the letter "F," rearranging rings on spindles to match a sample, sorting cards into color or number categories, recalling the locations of shapes in a two-dimensional matrix, or detecting X from O in letter sequences? The disconnection between tasks used to assess and build models of EF and what EF is used for in daily human life is a stunning chasm. The chasm cries out for a bridge, and that potential bridge is the concept of the extended phenotype as described above. The features of the extended phenotype model of EF help explain the nature and meaning of PFC/EF system injuries, disorders, or other impairments as discussed next.

Understanding the Effects of Injury, Disorder, or Impairment to the EF/SR System

This model of EF explains how socially and personally devastating injuries to or maldevelopment of the EF system (largely the PFC) are for long-term human welfare. First, such injuries or disorders can devastate the two developmental processes that give rise to EF itself: the self-direction of human actions for self-regulation across time to attain goals and the internalization of those self-directed actions. Even if these basic processes are spared, or developed normally, later injuries or disorders can still have direct adverse effects on any or all of the six Instrumental EF components: self-awareness; self-restraint; self-directed sensory–motor actions for mental simulation and ideation; self-directed speech and verbal thinking; self-regulation of emotion along with self-regulation of motivational states needed to pursue goals; and self-play or the creative component of goal-directed problem solving and innovation. What might this lead to? Well, depending on the component that is impaired, one could see:

• Impaired self-awareness, self-monitoring, and even an impaired general sense of self.

• A deficient ability to create imaginary constructions of the world, one's actions within it, and the consequences for those actions. Private simulation of event–response–outcome scenarios would be perverted or precluded altogether. Hindsight, foresight, and a sense of self-across time would likewise be defective. This would leave an individual with less or no ability to contemplate the future or would let him do so only at much shorter time horizons with a narrower temporal window onto that future. The individual would suffer a temporal myopia, being able to contemplate and prepare for future events only at close temporal range or only when they are imminent or have arrived in the temporal now. If sufficiently severe, the individual becomes blind to time, living chiefly in the proximal "now." Moreover, the individual would be less capable of imitation and vicarious learning, of self-defense against social manipulation, less able to cope with social competition, and more likely to engage in social predation or parasitism.

• Disorder or destruction of the self-restraint component leaves one with the obvious problems of motor, verbal, cognitive, and emotional impulsivity. Behavior that is being contemplated cannot be kept private from others. The individual says or does what she thinks and feels in real time as she thinks and feels it. There is an inability to subordinate the immediate self-interests of the individual to others or to the individual's own long-term interests. This leads them to be characterized as selfish, impulsive, and irrational. Distractibility, or a failure to inhibit responses to task or goal- irrelevant events would likewise be expected. In short, the individual cannot delay gratification, a capacity central to civilized conduct and education.

• Disruption of the private self-directed speech component would leave an individual less able to use self-talk for self-guidance, for self-questioning or interrogation, for verbal problem solving, and even for verbal reasoning more generally. Since reading, listening, and viewing comprehension likewise depend on such private self-speech and its related capacity to hold verbal and visual information in mind, a cross-modal reduction in comprehension would be evident. Implicit in such a deficit is that individuals so affected would be less able or unable to adhere to moral codes framed in spoken or written language as a means of guiding ethical conduct.

• Disturbance of the emotion regulation component would lead to the impulsive expression of emotion, noted above. Also occurring would be a defective capacity for the top-down regulation of emotional states in the service of one's longer-term goals and welfare and in accord with the social expectations for that context. The five vectors in which emotional self-regulation can occur in the Gross modal model of emotion would all be jeopardized, including situation selection or modification, attention deployment, cognitive reappraisal, and response suppression or modification. A complete disconnection of this emotional appraisal system from the working memory systems discussed above (visual–spatial–motor and verbal) would lead to an inability to evaluate the contemplated future, one's actions, and their consequences; the evaluative component of EF is no longer linked to these other systems. Decision making concerning risk/benefit trade-offs would be impaired, as Damasio (1994, 1995) has described it in his somatic marker model of this network.

• Impairment to the self-motivation EF component would lead to individuals becoming highly dependent on external, immediate consequences and gratification to sustain their actions across time to complete tasks and goals. Absent these external motivators, sustained attention and persistence toward tasks and goals become erratic or short-lived.

• Should the self-play or reconstitutive component of the EF system be adversely affected, then one could expect a decline in verbal, nonverbal, and action fluency, as well as a decline in the capacity for problem solving and innovation during pursuit of a goal. The individual, faced with an obstacle to their goals, would fall back on more overlearned, automatic, or otherwise inadequate strategies or quit the pursuit of the goal entirely.

Such deficits are relatively easy to describe or predict as they are those classically associated with descriptions of PFC disturbance or injury. Worth noting, however, is that they were generated from this theory as predictions of deficits and not from mere amalgamations of lists of symptoms of PFC disorders. They arise from having specified the mechanisms involved in a theory of EF and its extended phenotypic effects and thus what one could expect to lose if those mechanisms are perverted, distorted, or completely lost. That they map nicely onto descriptions of PFC-disordered patients is a consequence that can be considered corroborative evidence of the theory.

Not anticipated by other models of EF, however, are those that arise from the extended phenotypic actions and effects of the initial Instrumental components of EF. As a hierarchically organized model, it makes obvious how impairments at lower EF levels may radiate upward to affect higher levels. Yet it also shows that deficits at higher levels need not always radiate downward to the detriment of lower-level functioning. For instance, individuals may not be capable of sustained cooperative ventures (acting as a social unity or group cooperative to attain a common goal in which all share) but may still be able to engage in social reciprocity and exchange. The radiating effects of disturbances at lower levels outward to later, higher levels of human functioning can also show how PFC/EF disorders can have adverse effects on many fields or domains of human functioning, such as ethics and morality, marriage and parenting, law, education, health maintenance, economic behavior (occupational functioning, financial management), transportation (driving), and community participation (politics and government). The impact that EF deficits may have on traditional neuropsychological tests are trivial in comparison to those occurring at higher levels of the extended EF phenotype.

Viewing disorders of EF as an extended phenotype with hierarchically organized levels leads to the assertion that EF deficits, when sufficiently serious, can cause a collapse in the hierarchy from the higher to lower levels (or an outward to inward contraction of the concentric rings of the EF phenotype). Such a contraction is dependent on the severity and localization of the adverse effect on PFC development and functioning. Disturbance or injury to the EF system will not only adversely affect one or more of the six Instrumental EF components, but will also cause a contraction across the eight developmental capacities that arise from EF and that characterize each level of this outwardly radiating model of EF effects at a distance. Specifically stated, these are:

• A *maturational contraction or perversion* such that the individual's behavior either comes to resemble that of a younger, less mature member of the species or reflects a bizarre and abnormal variation of the normal performance of the species.

• A *spatial contraction* in that the individual is less capable of using both rearrangements of the physical environment and of social entities that surround it in its quest for self-regulation over time to achieve goals.

• A *temporal contraction* in the individual's time horizon—a reduction in their capacity for foresight and thus in the length of the temporal period over which they can consciously contemplate the future and make preparations to act in anticipation of that future. Deficits in EF produce a nearsightedness to the future (a temporal myopia), making the individual relatively time blind and thus more focused on the now or near-term than should be the case for that individual's developmental stage. The individual with EF deficits is therefore likely to be governed more by external events within their immediate sensory fields than by mental (internal) representations concerning hindsight/foresight and the future more generally. Those mental representations can no longer serve to guide their behavior toward delayed consequences and future goals as would be the case in normal individuals of that age.

• An *inhibitory insufficiency*—the individual is less able to defer immediate actions and thus less able to contemplate a future, the choices they may have, and the longer-term goals that may be worth pursuing.

• A *motivational time preference contraction or reward discounting increase*—the individual shows a greater discounting of delayed rewards (values consequences less as a function of their delay) in choosing what goals and consequences to pursue and thus can be characterized as showing a high time preference or poor delay of gratification.

• A *behavioral complexity contraction*—a decrease in the length, complexity, and hierarchical nature of goal-directed behavior because the goals being pursued are nearer in time and because the behavior necessary to attain those goals is necessarily shorter in duration, less complex, and less in need of being hierarchically organized.

• An *abstract to concrete rule contraction*—with injury to the EF system, the capacity for the individual to use more abstract rules for self-governance contracts such that higher-level rules, such as ethics, laws, and regulations, may no longer have any governing influence over behavior. The individual comes to be guided by nearer-term, more concrete, and hence more selfish forms of rules (and morality).

• *A social complexity contraction*—the number of interactions needed with others and the number of others with whom the individual trades, reciprocates, and cooperates will contract. Since the goals pursued are immediate or near term, the need for and motivation to share and cooperate with others, particularly socially important ones, diminishes greatly or disappears entirely. The result is a highly selfish, impulsive, hedonistic, and even socially callous or psychopathic nature to the individual's conduct.

• *A cultural scaffolding collapse*—The defective EF system no longer allows the individual to acquire and capitalize on the information available in the culture as well as on the products, devices, and other means that culture can provide to assist with the individual's goal-directed actions, to extend those goals further ahead in time, and to bridge those larger temporal delays. In the young, this would represent as well a decreased responsiveness or sensitivity to pedagogy.

All of these contractions will result in a loss of freedom or self-determination and the dynamic and flexible quality that higher levels of EF contributed to human adaptation to the environment. That is because the EF system provided for four additional levels of universal Darwinism or evolution of information acquisition that are now jeopardized or lost in the individual. The development of each new level of universal Darwinism added an additional degree of freedom to the individual's options, choices, and actions—degrees of freedom now in jeopardy or lost due to injury or EF disorders. Those individuals with PFC injuries will be more at the mercy of the immediate environment, less free to contemplate and choose among various options for responding to events, less dynamic and capable of rapid adjustment to changes in environments, especially the social and cultural ones.

Such reductions in capacity and contractions in a hierarchy are not self-evident in other models of EF. Yet this model clearly shows that individuals with EF deficits will therefore show a retraction in the eight capacities that govern their behavior.

Furthermore, these adverse alterations will change the nature and source of information that governs the individual's behavior. Those sources will shift backward from internal to external, from the self to others, from the possible future to the temporal now, and from delayed gratification to immediate gratification. This will be evident in individuals being:

- Less able to regulate their behavior by internal representations concerning the future and their goals, and thus they are subject to being controlled more by external representations in the temporal now.
- Less able to rearrange the physical and social environment in support of their efforts at self-regulation across time toward goals.
- More under the socially manipulative influence of others (social predation or parasitism) and less able to regulate or govern their own behavior for their own welfare.
- More preoccupied or governed by events nearer in time than are other normal individuals of the same chronological age.
- More focused on and governed by consequences in the immediate context or near term rather than aiming behavior at larger or more socially important consequences that lie ahead across longer time spans (deferred gratification).

Such impairments in EF components, contractions in the EF hierarchy, and reductions in the EF capacities are evident in descriptions of patients with PFC injuries dating back to Phineas Gage, as discussed in Chapter 1, even if not worded in precisely this fashion. It is little wonder, then, that deficits in the EF/SR system, however they arise, can have significant, serious, and even devastating consequences for an individual's well-being, welfare, and even survival.

Lest it go unnoticed, there would also be ample evidence of such EF distortions or deficits in the reports and judgments of others about the individual and in the archival records pertaining to that individual going forward following the injury. These are predictable consequences at the Extended Utilitarian zone of the EF phenotype. They include the effects such EF deficits would produce on parenting and child care, as well as on transferring resources to offspring for their survival and general welfare.

The Problem of "Why EF?"

This is a different question from "What is EF?" "How does it work?" and "How do you measure it?" Yet a failure to answer it leaves us with only a partial understanding of EF. To answer the question, one must think of EF as a biological adaptation (or suite of adaptations) and consider the ultimate ends for which that adaptation evolved. An adaptation is a complex design with a purpose: it solves a problem or set of problems for the organism in the environmental niche in which it has evolved. For what ends does EF exist? What is it accomplishing? What problem(s) in human daily existence does this suite of mental mechanisms exist to solve?

EF exists to solve problems that arise in group living, especially individuals with whom we are unrelated (Barkley, 2001). Group living with nonkin poses significant problems and significant opportunities for exploitation as our species has gone about striving to survive, reproduce, and see to its welfare. The problems and opportunities EF arose to solve and exploit were social problems, making EF a social organ or as Dimond (1980) declared, the seat of our social intelligence.

Conclusions

In understanding EF as an extended phenotype having effects at a considerable temporal, spatial, and social distance from its initial level of functioning, I have attempted to synthesize the conceptualization of EF not only with other findings within neuropsychology, but with other fields of human knowledge, such as social psychology, education and pedagogy, ethics and morality, law, economics, and even politics and government. The common thread across these fields and of this initial attempt at consilience (Wilson, 1998) is the human sense of the future—foresight: the capacity to create imaginary constructions about a possible future for one's self in contrast to a current state and to use this sense to identify, plan, and then drive behavior toward those ends. If EF is a set of neuropsychological abilities that serve to direct and sustain action toward a goal, and if such goal-directed action is the starting point for other fields of knowledge, then a useful synthesis has been achieved. By highlighting this common thread and then tugging upon it, one can unite fields of knowledge pertinent to EF that appear superficially disparate. Through this attempt at a synthesis not only can a broader understanding of EF be obtained, but the contribution of EF to understanding these other important domains of human endeavors and other fields of human knowledge can be made explicit. This synthesis is neither definitive nor an end to the great conversation in the literatures about EF and its exceptionally important role in human life; it is a continuation. It is to be judged by its utility. Is it better than prior models at understanding the nature and importance of EF in human affairs? Does it better account for the deficits that are seen in patients with PFC/EF injuries or disorders than prior theories are able to do? Here I have tried to discuss the value of the extended phenotype view of EF for understanding those deficits. Does it better guide the clinical practices of assessment and treatment of EF and its deficits than those prior models? Next we address these latter questions—the value of this view for assessment and treatment.

10

Implications for Assessment
and Clinical Management
of Deficits
in Executive Functioning

The Problem of How to Assess EF

The fourth problem associated with EF noted in Chapter 1 that needs redress was how EF is to be assessed. If the term is not defined operationally, then anything goes; any measure or test can be declared to be executive in nature by mere assertion. But once we have an operational definition of EF and a theory of how it works, one can immediately see how and why EF tests fall short of the mark as devices for assessing EF. That is because they do not assess self-regulation directly; they are conducted over incredibly short time intervals and so miss the cross-temporal aspects of EF; they ignore any social purposes for which EF may have evolved; and they utterly fail to grasp the significance of social reciprocity, cooperation, mutualism, and culture in their construction. Dogmatic adherence to the psychometric tradition of understanding and assessing EF at its most basic cognitive level is grossly inadequate. It provides only a superficial evaluation of even the conventional phenotypic view of EF. It fails to capture entirely the multilevel, concentrically arranged, affectively/motivationally charged, socially important, and culturally facilitated nature of the extended phenotype of EF/SR in everyday human activities. Furthermore, the available evidence concerning the reliability and validity of these tests does not justify their entrenched place in making such important declarations about an individual's capacity for executive functioning and self-regulation or the likelihood of their being impaired in important domains of major life activities.

Implications of the Extended Phenotype Model for Assessment of EF

The extended phenotype model of EF clearly explains the basis for the frequent findings in the neuropsychology literature on EF that EF tests are related to a low and often nonsignificant degree with EF ratings, to observations of EF functioning in daily life activities, or to measures of impairment in major life activities. Such tests are relatively brief assessments of the Instrumental level of EF. They are otherwise poor at ascertaining the cross-temporal organization and self-regulation of behavior to attain future goals that is the essence of the metaconstruct of EF and commonplace in daily life. Even then, they also miss the largely social purposes that EF likely evolved to address.

In contrast, observations and rating scales of EF collected in ecologically naturalistic settings are more likely to be evaluating the Methodical (adaptive), Tactical, and Strategic levels of EF. With greater attention to their construction, they might even be able to capture the principled stage as well as the social aspects of each of these levels, which even current rating scales largely ignore. Even so, rating scales are closer to and more likely to predict deficits in EF observed in daily life activities and impairments in major domains of life activities likely to arise from those deficits, especially at the Tactical and Strategic level. Psychometric tests of EF assess a different, more elementary, cognitive, and short-term level of EF in moment-to-moment behavior over an hour or a few hours in clinical or lab settings. While they may be arguably most proximal to the moment-to-moment activities of the PFC, they are not necessarily the best means for assessing it or the best endophenotypes of EF for purposes of neuroimaging, molecular or behavioral genetic, or other scientific research purposes merely because they are psychometric in nature. Ratings of EF, in contrast, evaluate EF at the Methodical, Tactical, and to some extent Strategic levels of EF as they play out over days to weeks to months to years of human daily life activities. Such observations and ratings are therefore closer to the impairments in major life activities likely to arise from EF deficits and so correlate far more highly with measures of those impairments.

The purpose of the evaluation and the level of EF of interest should therefore dictate which form of measurement may be most appropriate and useful. Even then, multiple methods of evaluating EF and of considering its multilevel phenotypic nature are essential if a representative portrait of the individual's actual EF in daily life is to be obtained. For clinical evaluations in which the goal of the assessment is to ascertain EF in daily life activities in natural settings and to predict impairments that may arise therefrom, the evidence and the hierarchical model of EF make it clear that observations, ratings, the reports of others, and archival records of extended EF effects in natural settings will prove superior to tests of EF in accomplishing this goal. Yet it remains commonplace to find clinicians and clinical scientists disparaging such methods in favor of the lab psychometric battery when the evidence makes plain that it is the tests that are more deserving of such disparagement than the naturalistic assessment methods.

The extended phenotype model of EF indicates that the assessment of EF must be as multimethod and multilevel as the construct itself and as the concerns of a particular case may warrant. In some instances, evaluating all levels may be necessary, especially where severe and pervasive EF deficits are indicated by the initial presenting concerns about this patient. In other instances, milder degrees of EF difficulties suggested in the referral concerns or patient/family interviews may suggest that the evaluation be targeted at only higher levels of EF, such as the Tactical–Reciprocal, or Strategic–Cooperative levels. Moderate to serious PFC injuries or EF disorders would warrant evaluation of the Methodical–Self-Reliant or even Instrumental–Self-Directed levels should concerns about the patient exist concerning adaptive functioning, independence, and self-care. Evaluating EF from the vantage point of the extended phenotype model means collecting information on as many of the EF levels of the model as may be relevant to the particular individual. If damage or dysfunction is even more extensive, then the assessment of the Pre-Executive level may be in order so as to understand how the injury or disorder may have distorted, retarded, or caused the regression in the Instrumental EF level once those pre-executive functions became self-directed and internalized. Unlike the traditional psychometric approach to defining and evaluating EF, one size does not fit all. Methods must be chosen that are appropriate to each level of the model; at many levels, psychometric tests would not be available or appropriate for doing so. The evaluation of EF therefore should not focus on just one level (instrumental, or cognitive) as is traditionally the case of using psychometric batteries.

Pre-Executive Level

As just noted, information about even the Pre-Executive level may be as important to obtain as that at the upper EF levels and may even suggest why disturbances at the Instrumental EF level exist. For example, individuals who are color blind in their vision are likely to have just as much of a deficit in their capacity for mental visual imagery (Kosslyn, 1994), given that the latter (self-directed re-sensing) is founded on the former pre-EF brain function. Likewise, individuals with delayed motor development and coordination are likely to experience problems in their mental simulations of the same motor actions (Maruff, Wilson, Trebilcock, & Currie, 1999), again given that the latter self-directed action is based on the former pre-executive function. It is not a great leap of inference to suppose that this is also true for language problems, visual–spatial disabilities, impaired play, and even emotional dysregulation; any problems evident in the pre-EF level of these abilities will adversely affect that EF module based on them. A general principle might therefore be stated that across the instrumental EF, deficits in the pre-EF function that is being turned on and directed toward the self at the Instrumental level of EF will likewise pose difficulties for that EF as it emerges.

All of this is to say that evaluations of EF should not ignore relevant non-EF or pre-EF neuropsychological abilities; such evaluations may provide important information on the nature of the deficits in EF. The pre-EF level can be evaluated, of course, by traditional psychological tests and even by some behavioral-neurological exams of pre-EF abilities (verbal and nonverbal subscales of intelligence tests, other tests of language, spatial, and motor abilities, attention tests, memory tests, etc.). Interviews that focus on the individual's history and current functioning in these domains in their natural ecology, along with medical records pertaining to the existence of structural problems with the brain or peripheral sensory mechanisms, may also prove useful. Interviews with others who know the patient well will aid in corroborating the patient's complaints. Moreover, interviews and ratings of emotional disorders that may adversely impact the EF of emotional self-regulation also need to be considered for use in such evaluations as particular details of the case may warrant.

Instrumental–Self-Directed Level

The Instrumental–Self-Directed level of EF can likewise be evaluated through these same general means. It is here that EF test batteries (focusing on inhibition, nonverbal and verbal working memory, planning, problem solving, creativity/fluency/generativity, etc.) *may* have some role to play, though it is an arguable point. When used, their role needs to be a much diminished one from their current venerated stature in the field of neuropsychology in view of their limitations. Even if these tests can be said to be assessing certain cognitive aspects of EF at the Instrumental level, they can still be criticized for largely missing the social nature and purposes of these EF components; for assessing the cross-temporal regulation of behavior over exceptionally short ascertainment periods; for only superficially sampling the complexity and hierarchical nature of goal-directed behavior in natural settings; for not evaluating the self-regulation of emotion and motivation components of EF; and for missing the bidirectional flow between EF and culture that serves as scaffolding for the outward expansion of the EF extended phenotype. Supplementing the test battery with interviews of patients about their history and current functioning, as well as interviews with others who know them well concerning this same information, may partially compensate for the inherent limitations of the test battery. It is also here that more ecologically representative EF tasks can be used if desired, such as Grafman's analysis of social scripts (Grafman, 1995), the Six Elements Test (Wilson, Alderman, Burgess, Emslie, & Evans, 1996), or the multiple errands task (Alderman et al., 2003), among others (Burgess, 1997). These may yield additional (and more ecologically valid) information than would the EF test battery alone. But the current and near exclusive reliance on test batteries as the only approach to assessing EF is no longer justifiable and, from an extended phenotype view, myopic; in time it might eventually be considered as negligence.

Methodical–Self-Reliant Level

At the Methodical–Self-Reliant level, interviews and rating scales completed by patients and others who know them well can be used that evaluate self-reliant (adaptive) behavior, such as the Vineland Adaptive Behavior Inventory (Sparrow, Cicchetti, & Balla, 2005), the Adaptive Behavior Assessment System (Harrison & Oakland, 2003), or the Scales of Independent Behavior—Revised (Bruininks, Woodcock, Weatherman, & Hill, 1997). Such measures are often viewed as being applicable mainly to patients with widespread general intellectual or developmental delay (mental retardation or autistic spectrum disorders). But adaptive behavior scales and inventories may be just as appropriate for evaluating this level of EF, provided, of course, that information in the referral concerns or patient/family interview suggests it is a relevant level to evaluate in that case. Such rating scales or structured interviews, however, are evaluating the extended phenotypic effects of EF only into its first most temporally proximal zone of effects—the effectiveness of EF in meeting the demands for daily independent (self-reliant) existence. By themselves they will give an incomplete picture of the remaining extended phenotypic levels of EF.

Rating scales of EF can also be used to evaluate this Methodical–Self-Reliant level of the model that complement those measures of adaptive functioning discussed above and specifically evaluate the five dimensions of EF behavior occurring at this level. Two behavior rating scales of executive functioning for adults will prove useful at this and even higher levels (Tactical, Strategic). They are the Behavior Rating Inventory of Executive Functioning (BRIEF; Gioia et al., 2000; Roth et al., 2005) or the Barkley Deficits in Executive Functioning Scale (Barkley, 2011a; 2012b). Given that the BRIEF appears to have recruited supernormal standardization samples, care must be taken in interpreting comparisons to the norms as the scale might overidentify examinees as having EF deficits. The adult sample was cleansed of all adults with psychiatric, learning, neurological, and chronic medical disorders, those taking psychiatric medications, and adults without Internet access, for instance (Roth et al., 2005).

Tactical–Reciprocal and Strategic Cooperative Levels

The aforementioned rating scales may also provide a glimpse of the Tactical and possibly Strategic levels of the extended EF phenotype, provided that their item content targeted the self-regulatory behavior and social functioning occurring at these higher levels. Certainly, the EF rating scales discussed above overlap with the nature of EF behavior occurring at these higher social levels. Those scales can also be supplemented with measures more specifically targeting the social aspects of EF. Some of the adaptive behavior scales and inventories noted above do have subscales related to basic social behavior and skills that may be applicable to evaluating this level of EF. Other rating scales that target social skills in adults specifically could also be used, such as the Social Adjustment Scale—Self Report (Weissman, 2004; Weissman & Bothwell, 1976), the Social Functioning Scale (Birchwood, Smith, Cochrane, Wetton, & Copestake, 1990), and the Social Adaptive Self-Evaluation Scale (Bosc, Dubini, & Polin, 1997). The latter two scales were not standardized on a current sample of adults, thus precluding comparisons to recent norms. For children, the widely used Social Skills Rating Scale (Gresham

& Elliott, 2010) might be helpful. Again, this level can also be assessed in adults by interviews of the patient along with someone who knows them well, such as a family member or spouse/cohabiting partner. And certainly measures of moral development as well as the reports of others who know the patient well and the archival records of the individual's history of impairment can all speak to the impact of the injury or disorder on these levels and even the Principled–Mutualistic stage of the Strategic–Cooperative level.

Extended Utilitarian Zone

This zone of the extended phenotype model is actually a zone of impairments arising from extended EF deficits and reflects the proximal, intermediate, and longer term over which EF has had effects at a distance. It can be evaluated by the traditional means of examining impairment. Impairment refers to functional ineffectiveness, not to symptoms per se (Barkley, 2011b). It is therefore first assessed through interviews with patients and others who know them well concerning the individual's history of functioning in major domains of life activities, such as education, work, marriage, child-rearing, financial management, and driving. Second, the clinician can review prior archival records pertinent to the particular domains of impairment of interest in any given case, such as medical, psychiatric, employment, workmen's compensation, disability, military service, driving, criminal, educational, or other records that may speak to the degree of impairment present in the particular case. A third means to evaluate this domain is provided in the fourth edition of the *Diagnostic and Statistical Manual for Mental Disorders* (DSM-IV-TR; American Psychiatric Association, 2000). It provides two clinician-rated scales for determining impairment. These are the Global Assessment of Functioning scale and the more specific Social and Occupational Functioning Scale. But such devices are merely crude ways to quantify clinical impressions of impairment; they cannot be compared to normative information on a general population sample of adults. A fourth method is to employ rating scales of impairment. A few have norms for use with children besides the adaptive behavior inventories noted above, such as the face pages of the Child Behavior Checklist (Achenbach, 2001) and the Behavior Assessment System for Children–2 (Reynolds & Kamphaus, 2001). More recently, the Barkley Functional Impairment Scale–Children and Adolescents has been developed and normed on a large sample representative of 1,800 U.S. children ages 6–17 years that can be used for this purpose (Barkley, 2012c). For adults, the only scale to my knowledge evaluating impairment in psychosocial functioning (15 domains of major life activities) that has recent normative data on more than 1,200 U.S. adults is the Barkley Functional Impairment Scale (Barkley, 2011b).

The point of this discussion is not to review in detail potential assessment tools that clinicians may find useful in evaluating the multilevel nature of EF as an extended phenotype. Instead, it is to encourage clinicians and researchers to at least examine EF as a multilevel extended phenotype in their evaluations and research protocols. It is also to fire their imagination as to what other methods might best be used to capture this multilevel model. In view of all the information provided in this book, clinicians and researchers can no longer be content with simply evaluating EF at the rather myopic traditional psychometric level of EF using a test battery.

Assessments using EF tests as the sole means of evaluating EF may be substantially incomplete and highly inaccurate. And using EF tests alone as endophenotypes for neurobiological research on disorders may also prove to be equally limited. Ratings and observations of EF constructs have proven to be as or more useful endophenotypes in neuroimaging (Buckholtz et al., 2010) and molecular/behavioral genetic studies (Paloyelis, Asherson, Mehta, Faraone, & Kuntsi, 2010) than have EF tests. The situation may well warrant repeating earlier research that relied solely on EF tests using other measures of EF, such as rating scales, and viewing EF from the multileveled extended phenotypic model set forth here if a more complete and accurate portrayal of the nature of EF and its relationship to various disorders is to be obtained.

The debate about the best means of defining and assessing EF is not merely academic. Every workday in the United States, hundreds, if not thousands, of individuals are being assessed by traditional EF tests. This is being done not just to render clinical opinions about clinically referred patients and their likely impairments in daily life activities, but to make formal official determinations of the presence or absence of disabilities that may profoundly affect an individual's life and livelihood. For instance, students are given or denied accommodations or special educational services in educational settings; workers are given or denied workman's compensation or social security disability benefits; victims of accidents are accorded or denied insurance settlements; war veterans are granted or denied compensation and even rehabilitation programs; and the legally accused are granted or denied special considerations or judgments. These are only some of the widespread practices in which opinions about EF are being rendered solely on the basis of the results of psychometric tests purported to assess EF.

This situation is unconscionable, given the already substantial and growing body of evidence that these tests cannot serve this purpose. Neuropsychology has long since abandoned its initial purpose of localizing lesions in the brains of patients, having been replaced in this mission by the far more accurate forms of neuroimaging. In place of that purpose, it has taken on as one of its missions the assessment of brain–behavior relationships relevant to evaluating and predicting how well or poorly people function in important domains of everyday life activities, in this case those that involve EF. The available evidence, however, indicates that EF tests cannot serve this purpose as the sole means of evaluating EF. EF ratings, observations, structured interviews, and other means are proving superior to such tests if the intent of the clinical evaluation is predicting impairment. It is time that clinicians cease using EF tests alone as the standard for the evaluation of EF in clinical practice.

Implications for the Clinical Management of EF Deficits

As with the above section on assessment, my aim is not to discuss in detail the treatment of EF deficits. There is much information on that issue in the literature on neuropsychological (and cognitive) rehabilitation. The point is to encourage clinicians and clinical researchers to broaden their view of EF treatments beyond that suggested by the traditional psychometric view of EF to that of the extended phenotype, multilevel model of EF/SR. If EF deficits are viewed as specific cognitive difficulties with tasks such as card-sorting by categories and repeating digit sequences forwards and backwards, then rehabilitation would consist of retraining of these sets of skills and related abilities. More is to be gained by understanding that EF is SR and extends as a phenotype upward through a hierarchical structure of increasingly complex behavior and outward to involve increasingly larger social networks assisted by increasingly complex cultural scaffolding. The latter perspective involves deficits in the EF/SR dimensions of self-management to time, self-organization and problem solving, self-restraint, self-motivation, and self-regulation of emotion as suggested in recent rating scales of EF evaluating these levels (Barkley, 2011a). It also includes the social activities of dyadic reciprocity, social exchange, group cooperative ventures, and even community mutualism not evident at all in the cognitive view of EF. Efforts aimed at accommodating EF deficits in time management, self-organization and problem solving, self-restraint, self-motivation, and self-regulation of emotions would not arise from the cognitive model of EF, but they *would* spring from the extended phenotype model of EF/SR and its inclusion of daily adaptive and social spheres of EF functioning.

Another distinction between traditional EF models and the extended phenotype model relevant to treatment arises from their widely disparate views on the origin and purpose of EF. The traditional cognitive model sees EF as a catalog of mental modules that process various types of information. The modules then pass on their processed information to other modules, all of which appear to be routed and scheduled by some "central executive" that remains unspecified and yet directs the action. How does such a view lend itself to developing treatment recommendations for a patient with EF deficits? The extended phenotype view does lead to recommendations. The Instrumental EF represent pre-EF actions that have been *self-directed and internalized* over development (and evolution) to give rise to "mental" information that is being actively held in mind so as to guide behavior across time. All recommendations flow from acknowledging that, in those with EF deficits, the self-directed and internalized form of EF is weak or deficient and thus cannot govern behavior as well as others are able to do. Therefore, going backward in the developmental sequence, there is a need for greater reliance on external forms of overtly self-directed actions (e.g., out-loud verbal self-speech) and even a greater reliance on external props and prompts within the sensory fields to help facilitate self-regulation.

The psychometric view of EF sees the EF as mental modules passively processing information and exchanging it along pathways with other modules. The extended phenotype model sees EF as conscious, effortful, self-initiated, and self-directed activities that strive to modify otherwise automatic behavior so as to alter the likelihood of future consequences (longer-term goals and desires). It views these self-directed activities as largely comprising self-directed attention, self-restraint, sensory–motor action to the self using chiefly visual imagery, speech to the self, emotion to the self and self-motivation, and self-directed play making it crystal clear just what humans are doing to themselves when they engage in EF/SR. This view would encourage individuals wishing to further develop or rehabilitate their EF/SR to repeatedly practice: self-monitoring, self-stopping, seeing the future, saying the future, feeling the future, and playing with the future so as to effectively "plan and go" toward that future.

The extended phenotype view of EF argues that the problems posed for those with EF deficits in major life activities have more to do with not using what they know at critical points of performance in their natural environments than with not knowing what to do. In short, information is not self-regulation. Just knowing about self-regulation will not automatically translate into actual self-regulation. The EF system is largely a motor or performance system rather than a sensory processing system. It is a system in which what one knows (skills and knowledge) is applied to daily life across time. To use the knowledge one has acquired in life, one must stop impulsively responding to immediate events and pause the ongoing action. This pause permits the executive system to generate the mentally represented information that will be needed to guide a more appropriate response in that situation.

As I have discussed in detail elsewhere (Barkley, 1997b, 2006, 2010; Barkley et al., 2008), treatments for EF deficits, such as ADHD or PFC injuries, should focus on several key recommendations that stem from the self-regulatory extended phenotype model of EF. All of these will be most helpful when they assist with the performance of a particular behavior at the *point of performance* in the natural environments where and when such behavior should be performed. A corollary of this is that the further away in space and time a treatment is from this point of performance, the less effective it is likely to be in assisting with the management of EF deficits. Not only is assistance at the "point of performance" going to prove critical to treatment efficacy, but so is assistance with the time, timing, and timeliness of behavior, not just in the training of the behavior itself. If such assistance is summarily removed within a short period of time once the individual is performing the desired behavior, then maintenance of treatment effects will be unlikely. The value of treatment lies not only in eliciting behavior likely to already be in the individual's repertoire at the point of performance where its display is critical, but in maintaining the performance of that behavior over time in that natural setting.

Disorders of EF pose great consternation for the mental health, rehabilitation, and educational arenas of service because they create disorders mainly of performance rather than of knowledge or skills. Mental health and education professionals are more expert at conveying knowledge and skills—how to change and what to do; far fewer are expert in ways to engineer environments to facilitate performance—where and when to change. At the core of such problems is the vexing issue of just how one gets people to behave in ways that even they know may be good for them when they seem unlikely, unable, or unwilling to perform. Conveying more knowledge does not prove as helpful as altering the parameters associated with performing that behavior at its appropriate point of performance. Coupled with this is the realization that such changes in behavior are likely to be maintained only as long as those environmental adjustments or accommodations are as well. To expect otherwise would seem to approach the treatment of EF deficits with outdated or misguided assumptions about the essential nature of EF and its impairments.

Principles of EF Deficit Management

Some of the principles of EF deficit management that arise from the extended phenotype model are, briefly, as follows.

Externalize Information

If the process of regulating behavior by internally represented forms of information (working memory or the internalization of self-directed behavior) is impaired or delayed in those with EF deficits, then they will be best assisted by "externalizing" those forms of information. The provision of physical representations of that information will be needed in the setting at the point of performance. Since covert or private information is weak as a source of stimulus control, making that information overt and public may help strengthen control of behavior by that information. Make it physical outside of the individual, as it has to have been in earlier development. The internal forms of information generated by the executive system, if they have been generated at all, appear to be extraordinarily weak in their ability to control and sustain the behavior toward the future in those with EF deficits. Self-directed visual imagery, audition, covert self-speech, and the other covert re-sensing activities that form nonverbal working memory do not have sufficient power to control behavior in many EF disorders. That behavior remains largely under the control of the salient aspects of the immediate context.

The solution to this problem is not to nag those with EF difficulties to simply try harder or to remember what they are supposed to be working on or toward. Instead, the solution is to fill the immediate context with physical cues comparable to the internal counterparts that are proving so ineffective. In a sense, clinicians treating those with EF deficits must beat the environment at its own game. Whenever possible minimize sources of high-appealing distracters that may subvert, distort, or disrupt task-directed mentally represented information and the behavior it is guiding. In their place should be cues, prompts, and other forms of information that are just as salient and appealing and yet are directly associated with or an inherent part of the task to be accomplished. Such externalized information serves to cue the individual to do what they know.

If the rules that are understood to be operative during educational or occupational activities, for instance, do not seem to be controlling the patient's behavior, they should be externalized. They can be externalized by posting signs about the school or work environment and its rules and should have the person frequently refer to them. Having the person verbally self-state these rules aloud before and during individual work performances may also be helpful. One can also record these reminders on a cassette tape that the person listens to through an earphone while working. It is not the intention of this chapter to articulate the details of the many treatments that can be designed from this model. That is done in other textbooks. All I wish to do here is simply show the principle that underlies them—put external information around the person within their sensory fields to better guide their behavior in more appropriate activities. With the knowledge this model provides and a little ingenuity, many of these forms of internally represented information can be externalized for better management of the child or adult with EF deficits, as seen in ADHD for instance.

Externally Represent or Remove Gaps in Time

The organization of the individual's behavior both within and across time is one of the ultimate disabilities rendered by PFC injuries and other EF disorders. EF deficits create problems with time, timing, and timeliness of behavior such that they are to time what nearsightedness is to spatial vision. They create a temporal myopia in which the individual's behavior is governed even more than normal by events close to or within the temporal now and the immediate context rather than by internal information that pertains to longer-term, future events. This helps to understand why adults with EF deficits make the decisions they do, short-sighted as they seem to be to others around them. If one has little regard for future events, then much of one's behavior will be aimed at maximizing the immediate rewards and escaping from immediate hardships or aversive circumstances without concern for the delayed consequences of those actions. Those with deficient EF could be assisted by making time itself more externally represented and by reducing or eliminating gaps in time among the components of a behavioral contingency (event, response, outcome). Caregivers and others can also help to bridge such temporal gaps related to future events.

Another solution is to reduce or eliminate these problematic time-related elements of a task when feasible. The elements should be made more contiguous. Rather than tell the person that a project must be done over the next month, assist him with doing a step a day toward that eventual goal so that when the deadline arrives, the work has been done but done in small daily work periods with immediate feedback and incentives for doing so.

Externalize Motivation

The model also hypothesizes that a deficit will exist in internally generated and represented forms of motivation needed to drive goal-directed behavior. Complaining to these individuals about their lack of motivation (laziness), drive, willpower, or self-discipline will not suffice to correct the problem. Pulling back from assisting them to let the natural consequences occur—as if this will teach them a lesson that will correct their behavior—is likewise a recipe for disaster. Instead, artificial means of creating external sources of motivation must be arranged at the point of performance in the context in which the work or behavior is desired. For instance, artificial rewards, such as tokens, may be needed throughout the performance of a task or other goal-directed behavior when few or no immediate consequences are associated with that performance. For the person with EF deficits such artificial reward programs become what prosthetic devices are to the physically disabled—allowing them to perform more effectively in some tasks and settings with which they otherwise would have considerable difficulty. The motivational disability created by EF deficits makes such motivational prostheses essential for most children deficient in EF, and they can be useful with adults having EF deficits as well.

The methods of behavior modification are particularly well suited to achieving these ends. Many techniques exist within this form of treatment that can be applied to children and adults with EF deficits. What first needs to be recognized, as this model of EF stipulates, is that (1) internalized, self-generated forms of motivation are weak at initiating and sustaining goal-directed behavior; (2) externalized sources of motivation, often artificial, must be arranged within the context at the point of performance; and (3) these compensatory, prosthetic forms of motivation must be sustained for long periods. If the external motivation is removed, the behavior will not be further sustained, and the individual will regress to more erratic goal-directed behavior with less ability to sustain actions toward tasks and goals.

In general, there are two reasons to do behavior management for anyone: for informational training and for motivational sustaining. The informational training is done for individuals who have not yet acquired a skill. Once the skill is taught through behavioral or other pedagogical methods, those methods can be withdrawn and the behavior sustained presumably by contact with the natural contingencies. But in EF disorders the issue is not ignorance or lack of knowledge of a skill; the problems are with the skill's timing and execution at key points of performance and with the self-motivation needed to sustain the performance. Behavioral treatments can provide the motivational or behavior-sustaining assistance. Removing the external motivation after improvement in task performance will result in a loss of motivation and a return to the baseline state of limited self-motivation and an inability to sustain actions toward goals.

By equating EF with SR, and by viewing the SR of emotion as described by Gross as but a specific form of a more generalized process of SR, the extended phenotype model of EF illustrates at least five vectors through which EF/SR can influence goal-directed activities: situation selection, situation modification, attentional control/redirection, reappraisal, and response modification/suppression. In attempting to assist individuals with rehabilitating or at least compensating for their EF deficits, these five vectors offer opportunities in which clinicians can strive to improve such deficits. While this can be done by directly working with the patient, it is likely to be greatly assisted by advising caregivers or significant others to assist the individual with these five pathways of SR. Modifying the "point of performance" as discussed in more detail below readily fits into the situation modification vector of SR. Various cognitive-behavioral therapies may prove useful at the reappraisal pathway. The point here is not to map out all possible ways by which these five vectors of SR could be used to boost EF in those with EF deficits but to make clinicians cognizant that such pathways are available for doing so.

Related to this idea of motivational deficits accompanying EF disorders is the literature on self-regulatory strength and the resource pool of effort (willpower) associated with SR activities. There is an abundant literature on this topic that has been overlooked by neuropsychologists studying EF, yet it has a direct bearing on EF given that EF is viewed as SR. As nicely summarized by Bauer and Baumeister (2011), research indicates that each implementation of SR (and hence EF) across all types of SR (working memory, inhibition, planning, reasoning, problem solving, etc.) depletes this limited resource pool temporarily such that protracted SR may greatly deplete the available pool of effort. This can result in an individual being less capable of SR (EF) in subsequent situations or immediately succeeding time periods. They are thus more likely to experience problems or to fail outright in their efforts at EF/SR and resistance to immediate gratification. Such temporary depletions may be further exacerbated by stress, alcohol or other drug use, illness, or even low levels of blood glucose. Research also indicates what factors may serve to more rapidly replenish the resource pool. These include:

- Routine physical exercise.
- Taking 10-minute breaks periodically during SR strenuous situations.
- Relaxing or meditating for at least 3 minutes after such SR-exerting activities.
- Visualizing the rewards or outcomes while involved in EF/SR tasks.
- Arranging for periodic small rewards throughout the tasks for SR-demanding settings.
- Engaging in self-affirming statements of self-efficacy prior to and during such tasks.
- Generating positive emotions.
- Consuming glucose-rich beverages during the task.

Some research further suggests that the actual capacity of the resource pool may be boosted by routine physical exercise and by routine practicing of tasks involving self-regulation daily for two weeks. From the extended phenotype view of EF as SR, these findings from the psychological literature on SR are directly pertinent to EF and its disorders.

Intervene at the Point of Performance in Natural Settings

Given the above listed considerations, clinicians should likely reject most approaches to intervention for adults with EF deficits that do not involve helping patients with an active intervention at the point of performance and across the extended EF phenotypic levels that are impaired. Once per week counseling is unlikely to succeed with the patient with deficient EF without efforts to insert accommodations at key points of performance in natural settings to address the impaired domains of major life activities. This is not to say that extensive training or retraining at the Instrumental level of EF, as with working memory training, may not have some short-term benefits. Such practice has been shown to increase the likelihood of using EF/SR and of boosting the SR resource pool capacity in normal individuals, at least temporarily (Bauer & Baumeister, 2011).

An implication for the management of EF deficits from the extended phenotype theory is that only a treatment that can result in improvement or normalization of the underlying neurological and even genetic substrates of EF is likely to result in an improvement or normalization of the phenotypic deficits. To date, the only existing treatment that has any hope of achieving this end is medication, such as stimulants or nonstimulants like atomoxetine or guanfacine XR, that improve or normalize the neural substrates in the prefrontal regions and related networks that likely underlie some of these deficits, such as those associated with ADHD. Evidence to date suggests that this improvement or normalization in ADHD-related EF deficits may occur as a temporary consequence of active treatment with stimulant medication, yet only during the time course the medication remains within the brain. For instance, research shows that clinical improvement in behavior occurs in as many as 75–92% of those with ADHD and results in normalization of behavior in approximately 50–60% of these cases, on average. The model of EF developed here, then, implies that medication is not only a useful treatment approach for the management of certain EF deficits but may be a predominant treatment approach among those treatments currently available. That is because it is the only treatment known to date to produce such improvement/normalization rates, albeit temporarily, for ADHD-related EF deficits.

Approach EF Deficits as a Chronic Condition

The foregoing leads to a much more general implication of this extended phenotype model of EF: The approach taken to its management must be the same as that taken in the management of other chronic medical or psychiatric disabilities. Diabetes is an analogous condition to many forms of EF deficits. At the time of diagnosis, all involved must realize that there is currently no cure for the condition. Still, multiple means of treatment can provide symptomatic relief from the deleterious effects of the condition, including taking daily doses of medication and changing settings, tasks, and lifestyles. Immediately following diagnosis, the clinician works to educate the patient and family on the nature of the chronic disorder, and then designs and implements a treatment package for the condition. This package must be maintained over long periods to maintain the symptomatic relief that the treatments initially achieve. Ideally, the treatment package, so maintained, will reduce or eliminate the secondary consequences of leaving the condition unmanaged. However, each patient is different, and so is each instance of the chronic condition being treated. As a result, symptom breakthroughs and crises are likely to occur periodically over the course of treatment that may demand reintervention or the design and implementation of modified or entirely new treatment packages. Changes to the environment that may assist those with the disorder are not viewed as somehow correcting earlier faulty learning or leading to permanent improvements that can permit the treatments to be withdrawn. Instead, the more appropriate view of psychological treatment is one of designing a prosthetic social environment that allows the patient to better cope with and compensate for the disorder. Behavioral and other technologies used to assist people with EF deficits are akin to artificial limbs, hearing aids, wheelchairs, ramps, and other prostheses that reduce the handicapping impact of a disability and allow the individual greater access to and better performance of their major life activities. Those methods provide the additional social and cultural scaffolding around the person with EF deficits so that performance in that specific setting can be more effective.

Besides the above recommendations, three EF-based cognitive-behavioral training approaches related to the phenotype model of EF/SR have been recently developed, researched, and published in manual form for clinicians (Ramsay & Rostain, 2007; Safren, Perlman, Sprich, & Otto, 2005; Solanto, 2011; Solanto et al., 2010). All three focus on addressing the types of EF problems that are associated with adult ADHD, such as poor time management, self-organization, and emotional self-regulation (Barkley, 2011a). Yet they are just as applicable to other EF disorders with modifications for the specific EF deficits evident in any given case. All are related in one form or another to my earlier self-regulatory model of EF (and so tacitly, though not explicitly, to the extended phenotype model developed here). Their contents could easily be extended to many other patient groups where EF deficits are a concern sufficient to warrant the use of a psychosocial training program. These training programs adopt a view of EF that is more similar to the model proposed here than the traditional cognitive psychometric view of EF. They go far beyond simply exercising the cognitive components of EF often targeted in purely cognitive rehabilitation training programs. Instead, the focus is on skills that would have much more of an effect on the five dimensions of EF behavior discussed above for the adaptive–self-reliant and higher levels of EF in the present model (i.e., time management, self-organization, problem solving, emotional self-control, self-motivation, etc.).

Intervene at the Most Disrupted Level

Of further importance to intervention is the multileveled nature of EF/ SR proposed here and the need to intervene at those levels most disrupted or adversely affected by damage or disorder. For instance, deficits at the Instrumental–Self-Directed (or cognitive) level of EF might be dealt with by training in self-directed inhibition, imagery, audition, and speech, among others, that is often the focus of cognitive rehabilitation (often computer-based) training programs. Although these may boost the initial low capacity of the individual in their inhibition, nonverbal and verbal working memory, planning and problem-solving abilities among others, evidence suggests that these capacities may decline after treatment has ceased. Thus retraining may be needed periodically to sustain initial gains. Adverse effects at the Methodical–Self-Reliant level may need to focus more on helping individuals to reorganize their external environment to facilitate performance of EF, self-care, and general adaptive functioning at this level. This could also be facilitated and amplified by artificial devices such as digital memory recorders, computers, personal data assistants, or cell phones to which periodic prompts and reminders are sent, and other such environmental prostheses. Also, the cognitive-behavioral programs just discussed above may be particularly applicable to this level of EF deficits as they, too, focus on rearranging the physical and social environment to help facilitate and amplify EF/SR in specific settings. There is also the need to help patients deal with potential social parasitism or predation from others, perhaps through more direct supervision, closer or more highly supervised living arrangements, or, in extreme cases, making the person a ward of a normally functioning relative. Deficits at the Tactical and Strategic levels will likely require training and ongoing assistance with social skills, etiquette, emotional self-regulation in social settings, and other therapies aimed at the social nature of these levels (reciprocity, cooperation, mutualism). Legal assistance may also be periodically required to address problems with social contracting, obeying laws, and conforming one's actions more generally to regulatory rules in specific settings. It may also be needed to protect the individual from serious breaches of performance at these levels and even the Principled–Mutualistic stage, as needed. In short, deficits at each level need to be catalogued and interventions aimed at each level, resulting in the design of a prosthetic environment around the

EF-impaired individual that would not have been at all evident from a merely psychometrically based cognitive view of EF.

Conclusions

Hopefully, this book has shown that the extended phenotype model of EF has considerable merit and utility in understanding the nature of EF, as well as the assessment and treatment of EF deficits, than do alternative models. No theory is ever perfect as proposed, and that is surely true of the present theory. All one asks of a theory is that it serve as a useful, albeit time-limited, tool—a means to an end. That end is providing a better explanation for what may already be known and to suggest further hypotheses and implications than has heretofore been the case with alternative or prior theories. The standard for judging any theory is utility: Can it be useful in understanding the material world better than any prior explanation? Can it better serve us as we strive to improve our survival and welfare and those of our descendants? To paraphrase Durham (1991) on theorizing, one simply seeks to build a better ship that can be floated for a time, and from the results we can then build an even better ship. It is trial and error with retention and criticism—theories evolve. All one can ask of the extended phenotype theory of EF offered here is that it is an improvement—imperfect but temporarily useful.

References

Achenbach, T. M. (2001). *Child Behavior Checklist—Cross-Informant Version*. (Available from Thomas Achenbach, PhD, Child and Adolescent Psychiatry, Department of Psychiatry University of Vermont, 5 South Prospect Street, Burlington, VT 05401)

Alderman, N., Burgess, P. W., Knight, C., & Henman, C. (2003). Ecological validity of a simplified version of the multiple errands shopping test. *Journal of the International Neuropsychological Society, 9*, 31–44.

Alexander, M., & Stuss, D. (2000). Disorders of frontal lobe functioning. *Seminars in Neurology, 20*, 427–437.

American Psychiatric Association. (2000). *Diagnostic and statistical manual of mental disorders* (4th ed., text rev.). Washington, DC: Author.

Anderson, P. (2002). Assessment and development of executive function (EF) during childhood. *Child Neuropsychology, 8*, 71–82.

Anderson, V. (1998). Assessing executive functions in children: Biological, psychological, and developmental considerations. *Neuropsychological Rehabilitation, 8*, 319–349.

Anderson, V. A., Anderson, P., Northam, E., Jacobs, R., & Mikiewicz, O. (2002). Relationships between cognitive and behavioral measures of executive function in children with brain disease. *Child Neuropsychology, 8*, 231–240.

Andreou, P., Neale, B. M., Chen, W., Christiansen, H., Gabriels, I., Heise, A., et al. (2007). Reaction time performance in ADHD: Improvement under fast-incentive condition and familial effects. *Psychological Medicine, 37*, 1703–1715.

Antal, T., Ohtsuki, H., Wakeley, J., Taylor, P. D., & Nowak, M. A. (2009). Evolution of cooperation by phenotypic similarity. *Proceedings of the National Academy of Sciences, 106*, 8597–8600.

Axelrod, R. (1997). *The complexity of cooperation: Agent-based models of competition and collaboration.* Princeton, NJ: Princeton University Press.

Axelrod, R., & Hamilton, W. D. (1981). The evolution of cooperation. *Science, 211,* 1390–1396.

Baddeley, A. (1986). *Working memory.* Oxford, UK: Clarendon Press.

Baddeley, A. D., & Hitch, G. J. (1994). Developments in the concept of working memory. *Neuropsychology, 8,* 485–493.

Badre, D. (2008). Cognitive control, hierarchy, and the rostro-caudal organization of the frontal lobes. *Trends in Cognitive Sciences, 12,* 193–200.

Banich, M. T. (2009). Executive function: The search for an integrated account. *Current Directions in Psychological Science, 18,* 89–94.

Banks, T., Ninowski, J. E., Mash, E. J., & Semple, D. L. (2008). Parenting behavior and cognitions in a community sample of mothers with and without symptoms of attention-deficit/hyperactivity disorder. *Journal of Child and Family Studies, 17,* 28–43.

Barkley, R. A. (1997a). Inhibition, sustained attention, and executive functions: Constructing a unifying theory of ADHD. *Psychological Bulletin, 121,* 65–94.

Barkley, R. A. (1997b). *ADHD and the nature of self-control.* New York: Guilford Press.

Barkley, R. A. (2001). Executive functions and self-regulation: An evolutionary neuropsychological perspective. *Neuropsychology Review, 11,* 1–29.

Barkley, R.A. (2006). *Attention-deficit hyperactivity disorder: A handbook for diagnosis and treatment* (3rd ed.). New York: Guilford Press.

Barkley, R. A. (2010). *Taking charge of adult ADHD.* New York: Guilford Press.

Barkley, R. A. (2011a). *Barkley Deficits in Executive Functioning Scale.* New York: Guilford Press.

Barkley, R. A. (2011b). *Barkley Functional Impairment Scale.* New York: Guilford Press.

Barkley, R. A. (2012a). Distinguishing sluggish cognitive tempo from attention-deficit/hyperactivity disorder in adults. *Journal of Abnormal Psychology, 121,* in press.

Barkley, R. A. (2012b). *Barkley Deficits in Executive Functioning Scale—Children and Adolescents.* New York: Guilford Press.

Barkley, R. A. (2012c). *Barkley Functional Impairment Scale—Children and Adolescents.* New York: Guilford Press.

Barkley, R. A., & Fischer, M. (2011). Predicting impairment in occupational functioning in hyperactive children as adults: Self-reported executive function (EF) deficits vs. EF tests. *Developmental Neuropsychology, 36*(2), 137–161.

Barkley, R. A., & Murphy, K. R. (2010). Impairment in major life activities and adult ADHD: The predictive utility of executive function (EF) ratings vs. EF tests. *Archives of Clinical Neuropsychology, 25,* 157–173.

Barkley, R. A., & Murphy, K. R. (2011). The nature of executive function (EF) deficits in daily life activities in adults with ADHD and their relationship to EF tests. *Journal of Psychopathology and Behavioral Assessment, 33,* 137–158.

Barkley, R. A., Murphy, K. R., & Fischer, M. (2008). *ADHD in adults: What the science says.* New York: Guilford Press.

Barkow, J. H., Cosmides, L., & Tooby, J. (1992). *The adapted mind: Evolutionary psychology and the generation of culture.* New York: Oxford University Press.

Baron, I. S. (2004). *Neuropsychological evaluation of the child.* New York: Oxford University Press.

Barta, Z., McNamara, J. M., Huszar, D. B., & Taborsky, M. (2010). Cooperation among nonrelatives evolves by state-dependent generalized reciprocity. *Proceedings of the Royal Society: Biology, 278,* 843–848.

Bauer, I. M., & Baumeister, R. F. (2011). Self-regulatory strength. In K. D. Vohs & R. F. Baumeister (Eds.), *Handbook of self-regulation: Research, theory, and applications* (2nd ed., pp. 64–82). New York: Guilford Press.

Baumeister, R. F. (2005). *The cultural animal: Human nature, meaning, and the social life.* New York: Oxford University Press.

Bekhterev, V. M. (1905–1907). *Fundamentals of brain function.* St. Petersburg, Russia.

Best, J. R., Miller, P. H., & Jones, L. J. (2009). Executive functions after age 5: Changes and correlates. *Developmental Review, 29,* 180–200.

Bianchi, L. (1895). The functions of the frontal lobes. *Brain, 18,* 497–522.

Bianchi, L. (1922). *The mechanism of the brain and the function of the frontal lobes.* Edinburgh: Livingstone.

Biederman, J., Petty, C. R., Fried, R., Black, S., Faneuil, A., Doyle, A. E., et al. (2008). Discordance between psychometric testing and questionnaire-based definitions of executive function deficits in individuals with ADHD. *Journal of Attention Disorders, 12,* 92–102.

Biederman, J., Petty, C. R., Fried, R., Doyle, A. E., Mick, E., Aleardi, M., et al. (2007). Utility of an abbreviated questionnaire to identify individuals with ADHD at risk for functional impairments. *Journal of Psychiatric Research, 42,* 304–310.

Birchwood, M., Smith, J., Cochrane, R., Wetton, S., & Copestake, S. (1990). The Social Functioning Scale: The development and validation of a new scale of social adjustment for use in family intervention programmes with schizophrenic patients. *British Journal of Psychiatry, 157,* 853–859.

Blackmore, S. (1999). *The meme machine*. New York: Oxford University Press.

Bogod, N. M., Mateer, C. A., & MacDonald, S. W. S. (2003). Self-awareness after traumatic brain injury: A comparison of measures and their relationship to executive functions. *Journal of the International Neuropsychological Society, 9,* 450–458.

Boonstra, A. M., Oosterlaan, J., Sergeant, J. A., & Buitelaar, J. K. (2005). Executive functioning in adult ADHD: A meta-analytic review. *Psychological Medicine, 35,* 1097–1108.

Borkowski, J. G., & Burke, J. E. (1996). Theories, models, and measurements of excutive functioning: An information processing perspective. In G. R. Lyon & N. A. Krasnegor (Eds.), *Attention, memory, and executive functioning* (pp. 235–262). Baltimore: Brookes.

Bosc, M., Dubini, A., & Polin, V. (1997). Development and validation of a social functioning scale, the Social Adaptation Self-Evaluation Scale. *European Neuropsychopharmacology, 7*(Suppl.), S57–S70.

Botvinich, M. M. (2008). Hierachical models of behavior and prefrontal function. *Trends in Cognitive Sciences, 12,* 201–208.

Boulton, M. J., & Smith P. K. (1992). The social nature of play fighting and play chasing: Mechanisms and strategies underlying cooperation and compromise. In J. H. Barkow, L. Cosmides, & J. Tooby (Eds.), *The adapted mind: Evolutionary psychology and the generation of culture* (pp. 429–450). New York: Oxford University Press.

Bransford, J. D., & Stein, B. S. (1993). *The ideal problem solver*. New York: W. H. Freeman.

Bronowski, J. (1977). Human and animal languages. In *A sense of the future* (pp. 104–131). Cambridge, MA: MIT Press.

Brown, J. S., & Vincent, T. L. (2008). Evolution of cooperation with shares costs and benefits. *Proceedings of the Royal Society: Biological Sciences, 275,* 1985–1994.

Brown, T. E. (2006). The executive functions and attention deficit hyperactivity disorder: Implications of two conflicting views. *International Journal of Disability, Development, and Education, 53,* 35–46.

Bruininks, R., Woodcock, R., Weatherman, R., & Hill, B. (1997). *Scales of Independent Behavior—Revised*. Rolling Meadows, IL: Riverside.

Buckholtz, J. W., Treadway, M. T., Cowan, R. L., Woodward, N. D., Li, R., Ansari, M. S., et al. (2010). Dopaminergic network differences in human impulsivity. *Science, 329,* 532.

Burgess, P. W. (1997). Theory and methodology in executive function research. In P. Rabbitt (Ed.), *Methodology of frontal and executive function* (pp. 81–111). Hove, UK: Psychology Press.

Burgess, P. W., Alderman, N., Evans, J., Emslie, H., & Wilson, B. A. (1998). The ecological validity of tests of executive function. *Journal of the International Neuropsychological Society, 4,* 547–558.

Bush, G., Valera, E. M., & Seidman, L. J. (2005). Functional neuroimaging of attention-deficit/hyperactivity disorder: A review and suggested future directions. *Biological Psychiatry, 57,* 1273–1296.

Butterfield, E. C., & Albertson, L. R. (1995). On making cognitive theory more general and developmentally pertinent. In F. Weinert & W. Schneider (Eds.), *Research in memory development* (pp. 73–99). Hillsdale, NJ: Erlbaum.

Campbell, D. T. (1960). Blind variation and selective retention in creative thought as in other knowledge processes. *Psychological Review, 67,* 380–400.

Carlson, S. M., Moses, L. J., & Breton, C. (2002). How specific is the relation between executive function and theory of mind? Contributions of inhibitory control and working memory. *Infant and Child Development, 11,* 73–92.

Carruthers, P. (2002). Human creativity: Its cognitive basis, its evolution, and its connections with childhood pretence. *British Journal of the Philosophical Society, 53,* 225–249.

Carver, C. S., & Scheier, M. F. (2011). Self-regulation of action and affect. In K. D. Vohs & R. F. Baumeister (Eds.), *Handbook of self-regulation: Research, theory, and applications* (2nd ed., pp. 3–21). New York: Guilford Press.

Castellanos, F. X., & Tannock, R. (2002). Neuroscience of attention-deficit/hyperactivity disorder: The search for endophenotypes. *Nature Reviews: Neuroscience, 3,* 617–628.

Castellanos, X., Sonuga-Barke, E., Milham, M., & Tannock, R. (2006). Characterizing cognition in ADHD: Beyond executive dysfunction. *Trends in Cognitive Science, 10,* 117–123.

Chaytor, N., Schmitter-Edgecombe, M., & Burr, R. (2006). Improving the ecological validity of executive functioning assessment. *Archives of Clinical Neuropsychology, 21,* 217–227.

Chronis-Toscano, A., Raggi, V. L., Clarke, T. L., Rooney, M. E., Diaz, Y., & Pian, L. (2008). Associations between maternal attention-deficit/hyperactivity disorder symptoms and parenting. *Journal of Abnormal Child Psychology, 36,* 1237–1250.

Ciairano, S., Visu-Petra, L., & Settanni, M. (2007). Executive inhibitory control and cooperative behavior during early school years: A follow-up study. *Journal of Abnormal Child Psychology, 35,* 335–345.

Corbett, B. A., Constantine, L. J., Hendren, R., Rocke, D., & Ozonoff, S. (2009). Examining executive functioning in children with autism spectrum disorder, attention deficit hyperactivity disorder and typical development. *Psychiatry Research, 166,* 210–222.

Cosmides, L., & Tooby, J. (1992). Cognitive adaptations for social exchange. In J. H. Barkow, L. Cosmides, & J. Tooby (Eds.), *The adapted mind: Evolutionary psychology and the generation of culture* (pp. 163–228). New York: Oxford University Press.

Crone, E. A. (2009). Executive functions in adolescence: Inferences from brain and behavior. *Developmental Science, 12,* 825–830.

Damasio, A. R. (1994). *Descartes error: Emotion, reason, and the human brain.* New York: Grosset/Putnam.

Damasio, A. R. (1995). On some functions of the human prefrontal cortex. In J. Grafman, K. J. Holyoak, & F. Boller (Eds.), Structure and functions of the human prefrontal cortex. *Annals of the New York Academy of Sciences, 769,* 241–251.

Dawkins, R. (1976). *The selfish gene.* New York: Oxford University Press.

Dawkins, R. (1982). *The extended phenotype: The long reach of the gene.* New York: Oxford University Press.

Dawkins, R. (1987). *The blind watchmaker: Why the evidence for evolution reveals a universe without design.* New York: Norton.

Dawkins, R. (1996). *Climbing mount improbable.* New York: Norton.

Deacon, T. D. (1997). *The symbolic species: The co-evolution of language and the brain.* New York: Norton.

Della Sala, S., Gray, C., Spinnler, H., & Trivelli, C. (1998). Frontal lobe functioning in man: The riddle revisited. *Archives of Clinical Neuropsychology, 13,* 663–682.

Denckla, M. B. (1996). A theory and model of executive function: a neuropsychological perspective. In G. R. Lyon & N. A. Krasnegor (Eds.), *Attention, memory, and executive function* (pp. 263–278). Baltimore: Brookes.

Dennett, D. C. (1995). *Darwin's dangerous idea: Evolution and the meanings of life.* New York: Simon & Schuster.

Dennett, D. C. (2003). *Freedom evolves.* New York: Viking Press.

D'Esposito, M., Detre, J. A., Aguirre, G. K., Stallcup, M., Alsop, D. C., Tippet, L. L., et al. (1997). A functional MRI study of mental image generation. *Neuropsychologia, 35,* 725–730.

D'Esposito, M., Detre, J. A., Alsop, D. C., Shin, R. K., Atlas, S., & Grossman, M. (1995). The neural basis of the central executive system of working memory. *Nature, 378,* 279–281.

Diamond, A. (2000). Close interrelation of motor development and cognitive development and of the cerebellum and prefrontal cortex. *Developmental Psychology, 71,* 44–56.

Diaz, R. M., & Berk, L. E. (1992). *Private speech: From social interaction to self-regulation.* Mahwah, NJ: Erlbaum.

Diaz, R. M., Neal, C. J., and Amaya-Williams, M. (1990). The social origins of self-regulation. In L. C. Moll (Ed.), *Vygotsky and education: Instructional implications and applications of sociohistorical psychology* (pp. 127–154). New York: Cambridge University Press.

Dimond, S. J. (1980). *Neuropsychology: A textbook of systems and psychological functions of the human brain.* London: Butterworths.

Dodrill, C. B. (1997). Myths of neuropsychology. *The Clinical Neuropsychologist, 11*, 1–17.

Donald, M. (1991). *Origins of the Modern Mind: Three Stages in the Evolution of Culture and Cognition.* Cambridge, MA: Harvard University Press.

Donald, M. (1993). Precis of origins of the modern mind: Three stages in the evolution of culture and cognition. *The Behavioral and Brain Sciences, 16*, 737–791.

Dugatkin, L. A. (2000). *The imitation factor: Evolution beyond the gene.* New York: Free Press.

Duncan, J. (1986). Disorganization of behavior after frontal lobe damage. *Cognitive Neuropsychology, 2*, 271–290.

Durham, W. H. (1991). *Co-evolution: Genes, culture, and human diversity.* Stanford, CA: Stanford University Press.

Eisenberg, N., Smith, C. L., & Spinrad, T. L. (2011). Effortful control: Relations with emotion regulation, adjustment, and socialization in childhood. In K. D. Vohs & R. F. Baumeister (Eds.), *Handbook of self-regulation: Research, theory, and applications* (2nd ed., pp. 263–283). New York: Guilford Press.

Eslinger, P. J. (1996). Conceptualizing, describing, and measuring components of executive function: A summary. In G. R. Lyon & N. A. Krasnegor (Eds.), *Attention, memory, and executive function* (pp. 367–395). Baltimore: Brookes.

Etkin, A., Egner, T., Peraza, D. M., Kandel, E. R., & Hirsch, J. (2006). Resolving emotional conflict: A role for the rostral anterio cingulated cortex in modulating activity in the amygdala. *Neuron, 5*, 871–882.

Fedele, D. A., Hartung, C. M., Canu, W. H., & Wilkowski, B. M. (2010). Potential symptoms of ADHD for emerging adults. *Journal of Psychopathology and Behavioral Assessment, 32*, 385–396.

Fehr, E., & Gachter, S. (2000). Cooperation and punishment in public goods experiments. *American Economic Review, 90*, 980–994.

Fehr, E., & Schmidt, K. M. (1999). A theory of fairness, competition, and cooperation. *Quarterly Journal of Economics, 114*, 817–868.

Finkel, E. J., & Fitzsimons, G. M. (2011). The effects of social relationships on self-regulation. In K. D. Vohs & R. F. Baumeister (Eds.), *Handbook of self-regulation: Research, theory, and applications* (2nd ed., pp. 390–406). New York: Guilford Press.

Fishbach, A., & Converse, B. A. (2011). Identifying and battling temptation. In K. D. Vohs & R. F. Baumeister (Eds.), *Handbook of self-regulation: Research, theory, and applications* (2nd ed., pp. 244–260). New York: Guilford Press.

Fitzsimons, G. M., & Finkel, E. J. (2011). The effects of self-regulation on social relationships. In K. D. Vohs & R. F. Baumeister (Eds.), *Hand-

book of self-regulation: Research, theory, and applications (2nd ed., pp. 407–421). New York: Guilford Press.

Frazier, T. W., Demareem H. A., & Youngstrom, E. A. (2004). Meta-analysis of intellectual and neuropsychological test performance in attention-deficit/hyperactivity disorder. *Neuropsychology, 18,* 543–555.

Freeman, W., & Watts, J. W. (1941). Frontal lobes and consciousness of self. *Psychosomatic Medicine, 3,* 111–119.

Friedman, H. S., Tucker, J. S., Schwartz, J. E., Tomlinson-Keasey, C., Martin, L. R., Wingard, D. L., et al. (1995). Psychosocial and behavioral predictors of longevity: The aging and death of the "Termites." *American Psychologist, 50,* 69–78.

Friedman, N. P., Haberstick, B. C., Willcutt, E. G., Miyake, A., Young, S. E., Corley, R. P., et al. (2007). Greater attention problems during childhood predict poorer executive functioning in late adolescence. *Psychological Science, 18,* 893–900.

Fuster, J. M. (1989, 1997). *The prefrontal cortex.* New York: Raven.

Gachter, S., & Herrmann, B. (2009). Reciprocity, culture and human cooperation: Previous insights and a cross-cultural experiment. *Philosophical Transactions of the Royal Society: Biological Sciences, 364,* 791–806.

Gachter, S., Herrmann, B., & Thoni, C. (2010). Culture and cooperation. *Philosophical Transactions of the Royal Society: Biological Sciences, 365,* 2651–2661.

Gailliot, M. T., & Baumeister, R. F. (2007). The physiology of willpower: Linking blood glucose to self-control. *Personality and Social Psychology Review, 11,* 303–327.

Gazzaniga, M. S. (1998). *The mind's past.* Berkeley: University of California Press.

Gilden, D. L., & Hancock, H. (2007). Response variability in attention-deficit disorders. *Psychological Science, 18,* 796–802.

Gilotty, L., Kenworthy, L., Sirian, L., Black, D. O., & Wagner, A. E. (2002). Adaptive skills and executive function in autism spectrum disorders. *Child Neuropsychology, 8,* 241–248.

Gioia, G. A., Isquith, P. K., & Guy, S. C. (2001). Assessment of executive function in children with neuropsychological impairments. In R. Simeonsson & S. Rosenthal (Eds.), *Psychological and developmental assessment* (pp. 317–356). New York: Guilford Press.

Gioia, G. A., Isquith, P. K., Guy, S. C., & Kenworthy, L. (2000). *BRIEF: Behavior Rating Inventory of Executive Function—professional manual.* Odessa, FL: Psychological Assessment Resources.

Gioia, G. A., Isquith, P. K., Kenworthy, L., & Barton, R. M. (2002). Profiles of everyday executive function in acquired and developmental disorders. *Child Neuropsychology, 8,* 121–137.

Goldman-Rakic, P. S. (1995). Architecture of the prefrontal cortex and the central executive. In J. Grafman, K. J. Holyoak, & F. Boller (Eds.), Structure and functions of the human prefrontal cortex. *Annals of the New York Academy of Sciences, 769*, 71–83.

Gollwitzer, P. M., & Oettingen, G. (2011). Planning promotes goal striving. In K. D. Vohs & R. F. Baumeister (Eds.), *Handbook of self-regulation: Research, theory, and applications* (2nd ed., pp. 162–185). New York: Guilford Press.

Grafman, J. (1995). Similarities and distinctions among current models of prefrontal cortical functions. In J. Grafman, K. J. Holyoak, & F. Boller (Eds.), Structure and functions of the human prefrontal cortex. *Annals of the New York Academy of Sciences, 769*, 337–368.

Grattan, L. M., Bloomer, R. H., Archambault, F. X., & Eslinger, P. J. (1994). Cognitive flexibility and empathy after frontal lobe lesion. *Neuropsychiatry, Neuropsychology, and Behavioral Neurology, 7*, 251–259.

Gray, A. (1946) *The socialist tradition: From Moses to Marx*. London: Longmans, Green. (Reprinted by the Ludwig von Mises Institute, Auburn, AL)

Green, L., Fry, A. F., & Myerson, J. (1994). Discounting of delayed rewards: A life-span comparison. *Psychological Science, 5*, 33–36.

Green, L., Myerson, J., Lichtman, D., Rosen, S., & Fry, A. (1996). Temporal discounting in choice delayed rewards: The role of age and income. *Psychology and Aging, 11*, 79–84.

Gresham, F., & Elliott, S. N. (2010). *Social Skills Improvement System Rating Scales*. San Antonio, TX: Pearson Assessment.

Grodzinsky, G. M., & Diamond, R. (1992). Frontal lobe functioning in boys with attention-deficit hyperactivity disorders. *Developmental Neuropsychology, 8*, 427–445.

Gross, J. J. (1998). The emerging field of emotion regulation: An integrative review. *Review of General Psychology, 2*, 271–299.

Gross, J. J. (Ed.) (2007). *Handbook of emotion regulation*. New York: Guilford Press.

Hale, J. B., Reddy, L. A., Decker, S. L., Thompson, R., Henzel, J., Teodori, A., et al. (2009). Development and validation of an attention-deficit/hyperactivity disorder (ADHD) executive function and behavior rating screening battery. *Journal of Clinical and Experimental Neuropsychology, 31*, 897–912.

Harlow, J. M. (1848). Passage of an iron rod through the head. *Boston Medical and Surgical Journal, 39*, 389–393.

Harlow, J. M. (1868). Recovery from the passage of an iron rod through the head. *Publications of the Massachusetts Medical Society, 2*, 237–346.

Harrison, P. L., & Oakland, T. (2003). *Adaptive Behavior Assessment System* (2nd ed.). Minneapolis, MN: Pearson Assessment.

Hauser, M. (2006). *Moral minds: How nature designed our sense of right and wrong*. New York: HarperCollins.

Hayes, S. C. (1989). *Rule-governed behavior: Cognition, contingencies, and instructional control.* New York: Plenum.

Hayes, S. C., Gifford, E. V., & Ruckstuhl, L. E., Jr. (1996). In G. R. Lyon & N. A. Krasnegor (Eds.), *Attention, memory, and executive function* (pp. 279–305). Baltimore: Brookes.

Hazlitt, H. (1998). *The foundations of morality.* Irving-on-Hudson, NY: Foundation for Economic Education. (Original work published 1964)

Hervey, A. S., Epstein, J. N., & Curry, J. F. (2004). Neuropsychology of adults with attention-deficit/hyperactivity disorder: A meta-analytic review. *Neuropsychology, 18,* 495–503.

Herwig, E. (2010). Me, myself, and I: How the brain maintains a sense of self. *Scientific American,* August 11, 2010, 58–63.

Hess, H., & Thibault, P. (2009). Darwin and emotion expression. *American Psychologist, 64*(2), 120–128.

Hinshaw, S. P., Carte, E. T., Fan, C., Jassy, J. S., & Owen, E. B. (2007). Neuropsychological functioning of girls with attention-deficit/hyperactivity disorder followed prospectively into adolescence: Evidence for continuing deficits? *Neuropsychology, 21,* 263–273.

Hofmann, W., Friese, M., Schmeichel, B. J., & Baddeley, A. D. (2011). Working memory and self-regulation. In K. D. Vohs & R. F. Baumeister (Eds.), *Handbook of self-regulation: Research, theory, and applications* (2nd ed., pp. 204–225). New York: Guilford Press.

Houk, J. C., & Wise, S. P. (1995). Distributed modular architectures linking basal ganglia, cerebellum, and cerebral cortex: Their role in planning and controlling action. *Cerebral Cortex, 2,* 95–110.

Huizinga, M., Dolan, C. V., & van der Molen, M. W. (2006). Age-related change in executive function: Developmental trends and a latent variable analysis. *Neuropsychologia, 44,* 2017–2036.

Izard, C., Stark, K., Trentacosta, C., & Schultz, D. (2008). Beyond emotion regulation: Emotion utilization and adaptive functioning. *Child Development Perspectives, 2,* 156–163.

Janicki, M. G., & Krebs, D. L. (1998). Evolutionary approaches to culture. In C. Crawford & D. L. Krebs (Eds.), *Handbook of evolutionary psychology: Ideas, issues, and applications* (pp. 163–208). Mahwah, NJ: Erlbaum.

Jokela, M., Ferrie, J. E., & Kivimaki, M. (2009). Childhood problem behaviors and death by midlife: The British National Child Development Study. *Journal of the American Academy of Child and Adolescent Psychiatry, 48,* 19–24.

Jonsdottir, S., Bouma, A., Sergeant, J. A., & Scherder, E. J. A. (2006). Relationship between neuropsychological measures of executive function and behavioral measures of ADHD symptoms and comorbid behavior. *Archives of Clinical Neuropsychology, 21,* 383–394.

Joyner, K. B., Silver, C. H., & Stavinoha, P. L. (2009). Relationship between parenting stress and ratings of executive functioning in children with ADHD. *Journal of Psychoeducational Assessment, 27,* 452–464.

Kahneman, D. (2011). *Thinking, fast and slow.* New York: Farrar, Straus and Giroux.

Kelly, K. (2010). *The case for legalizing capitalism.* Auburn, AL: Mises Instititute.

Kelly, S. D., Iverson, J. M., Terranova, J., Niego, J., Hopkins, M., & Goldsmith, L. (2002). Putting language back in the body: Speech and gesture on three time frames. *Developmental Neuropsychology, 22,* 323–349.

Kertesz, A., Nadkarni, N., Davidson, W., & Thomas, A. W. (2000). The Frontal Lobe Inventory in the differential diagnosis of frontotemporal dementia. *Journal of the International Neuropsychological Society, 6,* 460–468.

Kofler, M. J., Rapport, M. D., Bolden, J., Sarver, D. E., Raiker, J. S., & Alderson, R. M. (2011). Working memory deficits and social problems in children with ADHD. *Journal of Abnormal Child Psychology, 39,* 805–817.

Koole, S. L., van Dillen, L. F., & Sheppes, G. (2011). The self-regulation of emotion. In K. D. Vohs & R. F. Baumeister (Eds.), *Handbook of self-regulation: Research, theory, and applications* (2nd ed., pp. 22–40). New York: Guilford Press.

Kosslyn, S. M. (1994). *Image and brain: The resolution of the imagery debate.* Cambridge, MA: MIT Press.

Krams, I., Berzins, A., Krama, T., Wheatcroft, D., Igaune, K., & Rantala, M. J. (2009). The increased risk of predation enhances cooperation. *Proceedings of the Royalty Society: Biological Sciences, 277,* 513–518.

Krebs, D. L. (1998). The evolution of moral behaviors. In C. Crawford & D. L. Krebs (Eds.), *Handbook of evolutionary psychology: Ideas, issues, and applications* (pp. 337–368). Mahwah, NJ: Erlbaum.

Leary, M. R., & Guadagno, J. (2011). The sociometer, self-esteem, and the regulation of interpersonal behavior. In K. D. Vohs & R. F. Baumeister (Eds.), *Handbook of self-regulation: Research, theory, and applications* (2nd ed., pp. 339–354). New York: Guilford Press.

Lehto, J. (1996). Are executive function tests dependent on working memory capacity? *Quarterly Journal of Experimental Psychology, 49,* 29–50.

Leimar, O., & Hammerstein, P. (2010). Cooperation for direct fitness benefits. *Philosophical Transactions of the Royal Society: Biological Sciences, 365,* 2619–2626.

Levin, H. S., Fletcher, J. M., Kufera, J. A., Harward, H., Lilly, M. A., Mendelsohn, D., et al. (1996). Dimensions of cognition measured by the Tower of London and other cognitive tasks in head-injured children and adolescents. *Developmental Neuropsychology, 12,* 17–34.

Lezak, M. D. (1995). *Neuropsychological assessment* (3rd ed.). New York: Oxford University Press.

Lezak, M. D. (2004). *Neuropsychological assessment* (4th ed.). New York: Oxford University Press.

Lhermitte, F., Pillon, B., & Serdaru, M. (1986). Human autonomy and the frontal lobes. Part I: Imitation and utilization behavior: A neuropsychological study of 75 patients. *Annals of Neurology, 19,* 326–334.

Livesay, J., Liebke, A., Samaras, M., & Stanley, A. (1996). Covert speech behavior during a silent language recitation task. *Perceptual and Motor Skills, 83,* 1355–1362.

Lumsden, C. J., & Wilson, E. O. (1982). Precis of Genes, Mind, and Culture. *Behavioral and Brain Sciences, 5,* 1–37.

Luria, A. R. (1966). *Higher cortical functions in man.* New York: Basic Books.

Luria, A. R. (1973). *The working brain.* New York: Basic Books.

Lyon, G. R., & Krasnegor, N. A. (Eds.). (1996). *Attention, memory, and executive function.* Baltimore: Brookes.

Mahone, E. M., Cirino, P., Cutting, L. E., Cerrone, P. M., Hagelthorn, K. M., Hiemenz, J. H., et al. (2002). Validity of the behavior rating inventory of executive function in children with ADHD and/or Tourette syndrome. *Archives of Clinical Neuropsychology, 17,* 635–655.

Mahone, E. M., & Hoffman, J. (2007). Behavior ratings of executive function among preschoolers with ADHD. *The Clinical Neuropsychologist, 21,* 569–586.

Mahone, E. M., Hagelthora, K. M., Cutting, L. E., Schuerholz, L. J., Pelletier, S. F., Rawlins, C., et al. (2002). Effects of IQ on executive function measures in children with ADHD. *Child Neuropsychology, 8,* 52–65.

Mangeot, S., Armstrong, K., Colvin, A. N., Yeates, K. O., & Taylor, H. G. (2002). Long-term executive function deficits in children with traumatic brain injuries: Assessment using the Behavior Rating Inventory of Executive Function (BRIEF). *Child Neuropsychology, 8,* 271–284.

Marchetta, N. D. J., Hurks, P. P. M., Krabbendam, L., & Jolles, J. (2008). Interference control, working memory, concept shifting, and verbal fluency in adults with attention-deficit/hyperactivity disorder (ADHD). *Neuropsychology, 22,* 74–84.

Mariani, M., & Barkley, R. A. (1997). Neuropsychological and academic functioning in preschool children with attention deficit hyperactivity disorder. *Developmental Neuropsychology, 13,* 111–129.

Martel, M., Nikolas, M., & Nigg, J. T. (2007). Executive functions in adolescents with ADHD. *Journal of the American Academy of Child and Adolescent Psychiatry, 46,* 1437–1444.

Maruff, P., Wilson, P., Trebilcock, M., and Currie, J. (1999). Abnormalities of imagined motor sequences in children with developmental coordination disorder. *Neuropsychologia, 37,* 1317–1324.

Maynard Smith, J., & Szathmary, E. (1999). *The origins of life: From birth of life to the origin of language.* New York: Oxford University Press.

McCabe, D. P., Rodeiger, H. L., McDaniel, M. A., Balota, D. A., & Hambrick, D. Z. (2010). The relationship between working memory capacity and executive functioning: Evidence for a common executive attention construct. *Neuropsychology, 24,* 222–243.

McCabe, K., Houser, D., Ryan, L., Smith, V., & Trouard, T. (2001). A functional imaging study of cooperation in two-person reciprocal exchange. *Proceedings of the National Academy of Sciences, 98,* 11832–11835.

McCullough, M. E., & Carter, E. C. (2011). Waiting, tolerating, and cooperating: Did religion evolve to prop up human's self-control abilities? In K. D. Vohs & R. F. Baumeister (Eds.), *Handbook of self-regulation: Research, theory, and applications* (2nd ed., pp. 422–437). New York: Guilford Press.

McCullough, M. E., & Willoughby, B. L. B. (2009). Religion, self-regulation, and self-control: Associations, explanations, and implications. *Psychological Bulletin, 135,* 69–93.

McRae, K., Ochsner, K. N., & Gross, J. J. (2011). The reason in passion: A social cognitive neuroscience approach. In K. D. Vohs & R. F. Baumeister (Eds.), *Handbook of self-regulation: Research, theory, and applications* (2nd ed., pp. 186–203). New York: Guilford Press.

Merriam-Webster. (1989). *The new Merriam-Webster dictionary.* Springfield, MA: Author.

Michod, R. E. (1999). *Darwinian dynamics: Evolutionary transitions in fitness and individuality.* Princeton, NJ: Princeton University Press.

Miller, E. K., & Cohen, J. D. (2001). An integrative theory of prefrontal cortex function. *Annual Review of Neuroscience, 24,* 167–202.

Miller, G. F. (1998). How mate choice shaped human nature: A review of sexual selection and human evolution. In C. Crawford & D. L. Krebs (Eds.), *Handbook of evolutionary psychology: Ideas, issues, and applications* (pp. 87–129). Mahwah, NJ: Erlbaum.

Mischel, W. (1983). Delay of gratification as process and as person variable in development. In D. Magnusson & U. L. Allen (Eds.), *Human development: An interactional perspective* (pp. 149–166). New York: Academic Press.

Mischel, W., & Ayduk, O. (2011). Willpower in a cognitive affective processing system: The dynamics of delay of gratification. In K. D. Vohs & R. F. Baumeister (Eds.), *Handbook of self-regulation: Research, theory, and applications* (2nd ed., pp. 83–105). New York: Guilford Press.

Mischel, W., Shoda, Y., & Peake, P. K. (1989). The nature of adolescent competencies predicted by preschool delay of gratification. *Journal of Personality and Social Psychology, 54,* 687–696.

Mischel, W., Shoda, Y., & Rodriguez, M. I. (1989). Delay of gratification in children. *Science, 244,* 933–938.

Mises, L. von (1990). *Human action: A treatise on economics* (3rd ed.). San Francisco: Laissez-Faire Books. (Original work published 1948)

Mitchell, M., & Miller, S. (2008). Executive functioning and observed versus self-reported measures of functional ability. *The Clinical Neuropsychologist, 22,* 471–479.

Miyake, A., Friedman, N. P., Emerson, M. J., Witzki, A. H., Howerter, A., & Wager, T. D. (2000). The unity and diversity of executive functions and their contributions to complex "frontal lobe" tasks: A latent variable analysis. *Cognitive Psychology, 41,* 49–100.

Murphy, K. R., Barkley, R. A., & Bush, T. (2001). Executive functioning and olfactory identification in young adults with attention deficit hyperactivity disorder, *Neuropsychology, 15,* 211–220.

Murray, C., & Johnston, C. (2006). Parenting in mothers with and without attention-deficit/hyperactivity disorder. *Journal of Abnormal Psychology, 115,* 51–61.

Murray, E. A. (2007). The amygdala, reward and emotion. *Trends in Cognitive Sciences, 11,* 489–497.

Neese, R., & Ellsworth, P. (2009). Evolution, emotions, and emotional disorders. *American Psychologist, 64*(2), 129–139.

Nigg, J. T., & Casey, B. J. (2005). An integrative theory of attention-deficit/ hyperactivity disorder based on the cognitive and affective neurosciences. *Development and Psychopathology, 17,* 765–806.

Nigg, J. T., Willcutt, E. G., Doyle, A. E., & Sonuga-Barke, J. S. (2005). Causal heterogeneity in attention-deficit/hyperactivity disorder: Do we need neuropsychologically impaired subtypes? *Biological Psychiatry, 57,* 1224–1230.

Ninowski, J. E., Mash, E. J., & Benzies, K. M. (2007). Symptoms of attention-deficit/hyperactivity disorder in first-time expectant women: Relations with parenting cognitions and behaviors. *Infant Mental Health Journal, 28,* 54–75.

Norman, D. A., & Shallice, T. (1986). Attention to action: Willed and automatic control of behavior. In R. J. Davidson, G. E. Schwartz, & D. Shapiro (Eds.), *Consciousness and self-regulation: Advances in research and theory* (Vol. 4, pp. 1–18). New York: Plenum Press.

Nowak, M. A. (2006). Five rules for the evolution of cooperation. *Science, 2006,* 1560–1563.

Ochsner, K. N., & Gross, J. J. (2005). The cognitive control of emotion. *Trends in Cognitive Science, 9,* 242–249.

Ochsner, K. N., & Gross, J. J. (2008). Cognitive emotion regulation: Insights from social cognitive and affective neuroscience. *Current Directions in Psychological Science, 17,* 153–158.

Ochsner, K. N., Ray, R. R., Hughes, B., McRae, K., Cooper, J. C., Weber,

J., et al. (2009). Bottom-up and top-down processes in emotion generation: Common and distinct neural mechanisms. *Psychological Science,*
20, 1322–1331.

Oosterlaan, J., Scheres, A., & Sergeant, J. A. (2005). Which executive functioning deficits are associated with ADH/HD, ODD/CD, and comorbid AD/HD+ODD/CD? *Journal of Abnormal Child Psychology, 33,*
69–85.

O'Shea, R., Poz, R., Michael, A., Berrios, G. E., Evans, J. J., & Rubinsztein,
J. S. (2010). Ecologically valid cognitive tests and everyday functioning
in euthymic bipolar disorder patients. *Journal of Affective Disorders,*
125, 336–340.

Paloyelis, Y., Asherson, P., Mehta, M. A., Faraone, S. V., & Kuntsi, J.
(2010). DAT1 and COMT effects on delay discounting and trait
impulsivity in male adolescents with attention deficit/hyperactivity
disorder and healthy controls. *Neuropsychopharmacology, 35*(12),
2414–2426.

Paloyelis, Y., Mehta, M. A., Kuntsi, J., & Asherson, P. (2007). Functional
MRI in ADHD: A systematic literature review. *Expert Reviews in*
Neurotherapeutics, 7, 1337–1356.

Papadopoulos, T. C., Panayiotou, G., Spanoudis, G., & Natsopoulos, D.
(2005). Evidence of poor planning in children with attention deficits.
Journal of Abnormal Child Psychology, 33, 611–623.

Pennington, B. F., & Ozonoff, S. (1996). Executive functions and developmental psychopathology. *Journal of Child Psychology and Psychiatry,*
37, 51–87.

Piatt, A. L., Fields, J. A., Paolo, A. M., & Troster, A. I. (1999). Action
(verb naming) fluency as an executive function measure: Convergent
and divergent evidence of validity. *Neuropsychologia, 27*, 1499–
1503.

Picton, T. W., Stuss, D. T., Shallice, T., Alexander, M. P., & Gillingham, S.
(2006). Keeping time: Effects of focal frontal lesions. *Neuropsycholo-*
gia, 44, 1195–1209.

Piekoff, Leonard. (1993). *Objectivism: The philosophy of Ayn Rand.* New
York: Meridian.

Pinker, S. (1994). *The language instinct: How the mind creates language.*
New York: Morrow.

Pinker, S. (2002). *The blank slate: The modern denial of human nature.*
New York: Viking Press.

Pinker, S., & Bloom, P. (1992). Natural language and natural selection. In
Barkow, J. H., Cosmides, L., & Tooby, J. (Eds.), *The adapted mind:*
Evolutionary psychology and the generation of culture (pp. 451–494).
New York: Oxford University Press.

Popper, K., & Eccles, J. (1977). *The self and its brain.* Berlin/London:
Springer-Verlag.

Pribram, K. H. (1973). The primate frontal cortex—executive of the brain. In K. H. Pribram & A. R. Luria (Eds.), *Psychophysiology of the frontal lobes* (pp. 293–314). New York: Academic Press.

Pribram, K. H. (1976). Executive functions of the frontal lobes. In T. Desiraju (Ed.), *Mechanisms in transmission of signals for conscious behaviour* (pp. 303–320). Amsterdam: Elsevier.

Rabbitt, P. (1997). Introduction: Methodologies and models in the study of executive function. In P. Rabbitt (Ed.), *Methodology of frontal and executive function* (pp. 1–38). Hove, UK: Psychology Press.

Rachlin, H., & Ranieri, A. (1992). Irrationality, impulsiveness, and selfishness as discount reversal effects. In G. Loewenstein & J. Elster (Eds.), *Choice over time* (pp. 93–118). New York: Sage.

Ramsay, J. R., & Rostain, A. L. (2007). *Cognitive behavioral therapy for adult ADHD: An integrative psychosocial and medical approach.* New York: Routledge.

Rapport, M. D., Alderson, R. M., Kofler, M. J., Sarver, D. E., Bolden, J., & Sims, V. (2008). Working memory deficits in boys with attention-deficit/hyperactivity disorder (ADHD): The contribution of central executive and subsystem processes. *Journal of Abnormal Child Psychology, 36,* 825–837.

Rawn, C. D., & Vohs, K. D. (2006). The importance of self-regulation for interpersonal functioning. In K. D. Vohs & E. J. Finkel (Eds.), *Self and relationships: Connecting intrapersonal and interpersonal processes* (pp. 15–31). New York: Guilford Press.

Ready, R. E., Stierman, L., & Paulsen, J. S. (2001). Ecological validity of neuropsychological and personality measures of executive functions. *The Clinical Neuropsychologist, 15,* 314–323.

Reeve, H. K. (1998). Acting for the good of others: Kinship and reciprocity with some new twists. In C. Crawford & D. L. Krebs (1998). *Handbook of evolutionary psychology: Ideas, issues and applications* (pp. 43–86). Mahwah, NJ: Erlbaum.

Reynolds, C., & Kamphaus, R. (2001). *Behavior Assessment System for Children–2.* Circle Pines, MN: American Guidance Service.

Rhodes, S., Coghill, D. R., & Matthews, K. (2005). Neuropsychological functioning in stimulant-naïve boys with hyperkinetic disorder. *Psychological Medicine, 35,* 1109–1120.

Richards, R. (1987). *Darwin and the emergence of evolutionary theories of mind and behavior.* Chicago: University of Chicago Press.

Ridley, Mark. (Ed.). (1996). *Evolution* (2nd ed.). Cambridge, MA: Blackwell Science.

Ridley, Mark. (2001). *The cooperative gene: How Mendel's demon explains the evolution of complex beings.* New York: Free Press.

Ridley, Matt. (1997). *The origins of virtue: Human instincts and the evolution of cooperation.* New York: Viking Press.

Ridley, Matt. (2003). *Nature via nurture: Genes, experience, and what makes us human.* New York: HarperCollins.

Ridley, Matt. (2010). *The rational optimist: How prosperity evolves.* New York: HarperCollins.

Rilling, J. R., Gutman, D. A., Zeh, T. R., Pagnoni, G., Berns, G. S., & Kilts, C. D. (2002). A neural basis for social cooperation. *Neuron, 35,* 395–405.

Rizzolatti, G., & Craighero, L. (2004), The mirror-neuron system. *Annual Review of Neuroscience, 27,* 169–192.

Rizzolatti, G., DiPellegrino, G., Fadiga, L., Fogassi, L., & Gallese, V. (1996) Premotor cortex and the recognition of motor actions. *Cognitive Brain Research, 3,* 131–141.

Robbins, T. W. (1996). Dissociating executive functions of the prefrontal cortex. *Philosophical Transactions of the Royal Society of London, 351,* 1463–1471.

Rossano, M. J. (2007). Supernaturalizing social life: Religion and the evolution of human cooperation. *Human Nature, 18,* 272–294.

Rossano, M. J. (2010). Making friends, making tools, and making symbols. *Current Anthropology, 51,* S89–S98.

Rossano, M. J. (2011). Cognitive control: Social evolution and emotional regulation. *Topics in Cognitive Science, 3,* 238–241.

Roth, R. M., Isquith, P. K., & Gioia, G. A. (2005). *Behavior Rating Inventory of Executive Function—Adult Version.* FL: Psychological Assessment Resources.

Rothbard, M. N. (2002). *The ethics of liberty.* New York: New York University Press.

Rueda, M. R., Posner, M. I., & Rothbard, M. K. (2011). Attentional control and self-regulation. In K. D. Vohs & R. F. Baumeister (Eds.), *Handbook of self-regulation: Research, theory, and applications* (2nd ed., pp. 284–299). New York: Guilford Press.

Rushworth, M. F. S., Behrens, T. E. J., Rudebeck, P. H., & Walton, M. E. (2007). Contrasting roles for cingulated and orbitofrontal cortex in decisions and social behavior. *Trends in Cognitive Sciences, 11,* 168–176.

Ryding, E., Bradvik, B., & Ingvar, D. H. (1996). Silent speech activates prefrontal cortical regions asymmetrically, as well as speech-related areas in the dominant hemisphere. *Brain and Language, 52,* 435–451.

Safren, S., Perlman, C., Sprich, S., & Otto, M. W. (2005). *Therapist guide to the mastery of your adult ADHD: A cognitive behavioral treatment program.* New York: Oxford University Press.

Saint-Cyr, J. A. (2003). Frontal-striatal circuit functions: Context, sequence, and consequence. *Journal of the International Neuropsychological Society, 9,* 103–127.

Scholnick, E. K., & Friedman, S. L. (1993). Planning in context: Developmental and situational characteristics. *International Journal of Behavioral Development, 16*, 145–167.

Schroeder, V. M., & Kelley, M. L. (2009). Associations between family environment, parenting practices, and executive functioning of children with and without ADHD. *Journal of Child and Family Studies, 18*, 227–235.

Seidman, L. J., Biederman, J., Valera, E. M., Monuteaux, M. C., Doyle, A. E., & Faraone, S. V. (2006). Neuropsychological functioning in girls with attention-deficit/hyperactivity disorder with and without learning disabilities. *Neuropsychology, 20*, 166–177.

Senn, T. E., Espy, K. A., & Kaufmann, P. M. (2004). Using path analysis to understand executive function organization in preschool children. *Developmental Neuropsychology, 26*, 445–464.

Sergeant, J. A., Geurts, H., & Oosterlaan, J. (2002). How specific is a deficit of executive functioning for attention-deficit/hyperactivity disorder? *Behavioral Brain Reviews, 130*, 3–28.

Shallice, T. (1982). Specific impairments in planning. *Philosophical Transactions of the Royal Society of London Series B. Biological Sciences, 298*, 199–209.

Shallice, T. (1990). *From neuropsychology to mental structure.* New York: Oxford University Press.

Shallice, T. (1994). Multiple levels of control processes. In C. Umilta & M. Moscovitch (Eds.), *Attention and performance XV* (pp. 395–420). Cambridge, MA: MIT Press.

Shallice, T., & Burgess, P. W. (1991). Deficits in strategy application following frontal lobe damage in man. *Brain, 114*, 727–741.

Shermer, M. (2011). Sacred salubriousness: Why religious belief is not the only path to a healthier life. *Scientific American, December,* 102.

Shiffer, J. E. (2011, February 6). Beware of dating-site scams. *Star Tribune,* Minneapolis, MN. (Reprinted in the *Post and Courier,* Charleston, SC, p. 15A)

Shute, G. E., & Huertas, V. (1990). Developmental variability in frontal lobe function. *Developmental Neuropsychology, 6*, 1–11.

Singer, B. D., & Bashir, A. S. (1999). What are executive functions and self-regulation and what do they have to do with language-learning disorders? *Language, Speech, and Hearing Services in Schools, 30*, 265–273.

Skinner, B. F. (1981). Selection by consequences. *Science, 213*, 501–504.

Skinner, B. F. (1984). Selection by consequences. *The Behavioral and Brain Sciences, 7*, 477–510.

Solanto, M. V. (2011). *Cognitive-Behavioral Therapy for Adult ADHD: Targeting Executive Dysfunction.* New York: Guilford Press.

Solanto, M. V., Marks, D. J., Wasserstein, J., Mitchell, K., Abikoff, H., Alvir, J. M. J., & Kofman, M. D. (2010). Efficacy of meta-cognitive therapy for adult ADHD. *American Journal of Psychiatry, 167*, 958–968.

Sparrow, S. S., Cicchetti, D. V., & Balla, D. A. (2005). *The Vineland Adaptive Behavior Scale—Second Edition*. Minneapolis, MN: Pearson Assessment.

Stavro, G. M., Ettenhofer, M. L., & Nigg, J. T. (2007). Executive functions and adaptive functioning in young adults with attention-deficit/hyperactivity disorder. *Journal of the International Neuropsychological Society, 13,* 324–334.

Stuss, D. T. (1992). Biological and psychological development of executive functions. *Brain and Cognition, 20*(1), 8–23.

Stuss, D., & Alexander, M. (2000). Executive functions and the frontal lobes: A conceptual view. *Psychological Research, 63,* 289–298.

Stuss, D. T., & Benson, D. F. (1986). *The frontal lobes*. New York: Raven Press.

Suzuki, S., Niki, K., Fujisaki, S., & Akiyama, E. (2011). Neural basis of conditional cooperation. *Social Cognitive and Affective Neuroscience, 6,* 338–347.

Swensen, A. R., Allen, A. J., Kruesi, M. P., Buesching, D. P., & Goldberg, G. (2004). *Risk of premature death from misadventure in patients with attention-deficit/hyperactivity disorder*. Unpublished manuscript, Eli Lilly Co., Indianapolis, IN.

Symons, D. (1992). On the use and misuse of Darwinism in the study of human behavior. In J. H. Barkow, L. Cosmides, & J. Tooby (Eds.), *The adapted mind: Evolutionary psychology and the generation of culture* (pp. 137–161). New York: Oxford University Press.

Taylor, T. (2010). *The artificial ape: How technology changed the course of human evolution*. New York: Palgrave Macmillan.

Thorell, L. B., & Nyberg, L. (2008). The Childhood Executive Functioning Inventory (CHEXI): A new rating instrument for parents and teachers. *Developmental Neuropsychology, 33,* 536–552.

Tooby, J., & Cosmides, L. (1992). The psychological foundations of culture. In J. H. Barkow, L. Cosmides, & J. Tooby (Eds.), *The adapted mind: Evolutionary psychology and the generation of culture* (pp. 19–136). New York: Oxford University Press.

Valera, E. M., Faraone, S. V., Murray, K. E., & Seidman, L. J. (2007). Meta-analysis of structural imaging findings in attention-deficit/hyperactivity disorder. *Biological Psychiatry, 61,* 1361–1369.

van Leeuwen, M. J., van Baaren, R. B., Martin, D., Dijksterhuis, A., & Bekkering, H. (2009). Executive functioning and imitation: Increasing working memory load facilitates behavioural imitation. *Neuropsychologia, 47,* 3265–3270.

Vazsonyi, A. T., & Huang, L. (2010). Where self-control comes from: On the development of self-control and its relationship to deviance over time. *Developmental Psychology, 46,* 245–257.

Vriezen, E. R., & Pigott, S. E. (2002). The relationship between parental report on the BRIEF and performance-based measures of executive function in children with moderate to severe traumatic brain injury. *Child Neuropsychology, 8,* 296–303.

Vygotsky, L. S. (1962). *Thought and language* (E. Hanfmann & G. Vakar, Eds. & Trans.). Cambridge, MA: MIT Press.

Vygotsky, L. S. (1978). *Mind and society.* Cambridge, MA: Harvard University Press.

Vygotsky, L. S. (1987). Thinking and speech. In *The collected works of L. S. Vygotsky: Vol. 1. Problems in general psychology* (N. Minich, Trans., pp. 37–285). New York: Plenum.

Wagner, D. D., & Heatherington, T. F. (2011). Giving in to temptation: The emerging cognitive neuroscience of self-regulatory failure. In K. D. Vohs & R. F. Baumeister (Eds.), *Handbook of self-regulation: Research, theory, and applications* (2nd ed., pp. 41–63). New York: Guilford Press.

Wahlsted, C., Thorell, L. B., & Bohlin, G. (2008). ADHD symptoms and executive function impairment: Early predictors of later behavioral problems. *Developmental Neuropsychology, 33,* 160–178.

Watson, S. J., & Mash, E. J. (in press). The relationship between symptoms of attention-deficit/hyperactivity disorder and self-reported parental cognitions and behaviors in mothers of young infants. *Journal of Reproductive and Infant Psychology.*

Weissman, M. M. (2004). *Social Adjustment Scale—Self-Report.* North Tonawanda, NY: Multi-Health Systems.

Weissman, M. M., & Bothwell, S. (1976). Assessment of social adjustment by patient self-report. *Archives of General Psychiatry, 33,* 1111–1115.

Welsh, M. C. (2002). Developmental and clinical variations in executive functions. In D. L. Molfese & V. J. Molfese (Eds.), *Developmental variations in learning: Applications to social, executive function, language, and reading skills* (pp. 139–185). Mahwah, NJ: Erlbaum.

Welsh, M. C., & Pennington, B. F. (1988). Assessing frontal lobe functioning in children: Views from developmental psychology. *Developmental Neuropsychology, 4,* 199–230.

Wheeler, M. A., Stuss, D. T., & Tulving, E. (1997). Toward a theory of episodic memory: The frontal lobes and autonoetic consciousness. *Psychological Bulletin, 121,* 331–354.

Wilding, J. (2005). Is attention impaired in ADHD? *British Journal of Developmental Psychology, 23,* 487–505.

Wilens, T. E., Martelon, M., Fried, R., Petty, C., Bateman, C., & Biederman, J. (2011). Do executive function deficits predict later substance use disorders among adolescents and young adults? *Journal of the American Academy of Child and Adolescent Psychiatry, 50,* 141–149.

Willcutt, E. G., Doyle, A. E., Nigg, J. T., Faraone, S. V., & Pennington, B. F. (2005). Validity of the executive function theory of attention-deficit/

hyperactivity disorder: A meta-analytic review. *Biological Psychiatry, 57,* 1336–1346.

Wilson, B. A., Alderman, N., Burgess, P. W., Emslie, H., & Evans, J. J. (1996). *Behavioral Assessment of the Dysexecutive Syndrome.* Bury St. Edmonds, UK: Thames Valley Test Company.

Wilson, E. O. (1998). *Consilience: The unity of knowledge.* New York: Knopf.

Wolf, L. E., & Wasserstein, J. (2001). Adult ADHD: Concluding thoughts. In J. Wasserstein, L. E. Wolf, & F. F. Lefever (Eds.), Adult attention deficit hyperactivity disorder: Brain mechanisms and life outcomes. *Annals of the New York Academy of Sciences, 931,* 396–408.

Wood, R. L. I., & Liossi, C. (2006). The ecological validity of executive function tests in a severely brain injured sample. *Archives of Clinical Neuropsychology, 21,* 429–437.

Wozniak, R. (2009). Consciousness, social heredity, and development: The evolutionary thought of James Mark Baldwin. *American Psychologist, 62*(2), 93–101.

Wright, R. (1994). *The moral animal—Why we are the way we are: The new science of evolutionary psychology.* New York: Vintage Books.

Wright, R. (2000). *Nonzero: The logic of human destiny.* New York: Vintage Books.

Zahavi, Amotz, & Zahavi, Avishag. (1997). *The handicap principle: A missing piece of Darwin's puzzle.* New York: Oxford University Press.

Zandt, F., Prior, M., & Kyrios, M. (2009). Similarities and differences between children and adolescents with autism spectrum disorder and those with obsessive compulsive disorder: Executive functioning and repetitive behavior. *Autism, 13,* 43–57.

Zelazo, P. D., Muller, U., Frye, D., & Marcovitch, S. (2003). The development of executive function: Cognitive complexity and control—revised. *Monographs of the Society for Research in Child Development, 68*(3), 93–119.

Index

Inanimate artifacts
  genes extended phenotype evolvement,
    39–41
    cooperative sharing, 41–43
  evolutionary level, 53, 58
Incomplete theories, EF problem, 177–188
Information encoding, in evolution
    algorithm, 54
Information-processing theory of
    Borkowski and Burke, 18–19
Information updating, EF factor analysis,
    22
Inhibition. See also Inhibitory capacity
  evolutionary and developmental
    considerations, 102
  fractional future sense, 85
  Instrumental–Self-Directed EF level,
    81–82, 105
  Self-restraint creation function, 174
Inhibitory capacity, 70
  developmental EF goal, 70
  Instrumental–Self-Directed level, 105
  Methodical–Self-Reliant level, 122
  insufficiency effect, 185
  interactions, 70
  Tactical–Reciprocal level, 141
Injuries. See Prefrontal cortex injuries/
    disorders
Innovation
  cultural aspects, 74–75
  extended EF phenotype, 73–75
  and vicarious learning, 74–75
Insects. See Social insects
Instrumental Self-Directed EF level,
    79–107
  assessment/evaluation, 193–194
  awareness of self across time, 85–86
  components, 79–92, 177–178
    necessity, 95–96
  developmental considerations, 102–103
  emerging developmental capacities,
    104–107
  evolutionary considerations, 102–103
  executive inhibition, 81–82
  extended EF phenotype, 104, 105f,
    177–178
  goal attainment, 64–65
  internalization of speech process, 79–80
  internalized mental processes, 63
  Pre-Executive level use, 77
  prefrontal cortex disorders, 184
  self-awareness actions, 81
  self-directed appraisal, 87–90

self-directed play, 90–92
self-directed private speech, 86–87
self-directed sensory–motor action,
    82–86
self-direction, 63, 65, 79–80
self-regulatory actions, 81–92
self-restraint, 81–82
  social significance, 65
  three components necessity, 95–96
Insurance risk pool, 130
Intentionality, versus computers, 27
Internalization
  executive functioning component, 82
  extended EF phenotype property, 181
  Instrumental–Self-Directed EF level, 80
  sensory–motor actions, 84
Internalization of speech, function, 86–87
Intervention
  chronic conditions approach, 206–208
  deficit management principles, 201–209
  externalized information, 201–202
  externalized motivation, 203–205
  most disruptive level, 208–209
  point of performance, 205–206
  time problems, 202–203
Interviews, zone of impairments, 196–197
Intraspecies competition
  plagiarism and, 117
  self-reliance level and, 114
IQ, psychomotor tests validity, 11

J

Joint cooperation, 147–148
Judgments of others, 166

K

Kin selection, reciprocity, 128–130

L

Language
  behavior effects without host invasion,
    46
  evolutionary emergence, 102–103
  visual imagery stepping stone, 102
Law, executive functioning, 179–180
Leisure and labor distinction, 96
Levels, 60
  executive functioning, 63–68
  Pre-Executive functions, 75–78
Limited resource pool, and self-regulation,
    94–95
Locomotion, animals versus computers, 27